PLUCKED

PLUCKED

A History of Hair Removal

REBECCA M. HERZIG

NEW YORK UNIVERSITY PRESS

New York and London

NEW YORK UNIVERSITY PRESS
New York and London
www.nyupress.org

References to Internet websites (URLs) were accurate at the time of writing.
Neither the author nor New York University Press is responsible for URLs that
may have expired or changed since the manuscript was prepared.

Library of Congress Cataloging-in-Publication Data
Herzig, Rebecca M., 1971-
Plucked : a history of hair removal / Rebecca M. Herzig.
pages cm
Includes bibliographical references and index.
ISBN 978-1-4798-4082-3 (hardback)
1. Hair—Removal—United States—History. 2. Hair—Social aspects—United
States—History. 3. Body hair—Social aspects—United States—History. 4. Human
body—Social aspects—United States—History. I. Title.
RL92.H49 2015
617.4'779—dc23
2014027535

New York University Press books are printed on acid-free paper,
and their binding materials are chosen for strength and durability.
We strive to use environmentally responsible suppliers and materials
to the greatest extent possible in publishing our books.

Manufactured in the United States of America

10 9 8 7 6 5 4 3 2 1

Also available as an ebook

For Jill Hopkins Herzig

Contents

INTRODUCTION: NECESSARY SUFFERING

IN THE CLOSING months of 2006, representatives of the International Committee of the Red Cross (ICRC) traveled to the internment facility at Guantánamo Bay run by the U.S. Department of Defense. There, the representatives conducted private interviews with fourteen "high value" detainees held in custody by the U.S. Central Intelligence Agency (CIA), in accordance with the ICRC's legal obligation to monitor compliance with the Geneva Conventions. Their resulting forty-page report on detainee treatment, sent to the acting general counsel of the CIA in February 2007, concluded that the "totality of circumstances" in which the detainees were held "amounted to an arbitrary deprivation of liberty." Other aspects of the detention program "constituted cruel, inhuman or degrading treatment," while "in many cases" the combined treatments to which the detainees were subjected "constituted torture."[1] The report devoted a separate discussion to each of the "main elements" of detainee abuse, including beating and kicking, prolonged shackling, confinement in a box, and deprivation of food.

Listed among these elements of abuse was another category: hair removal—or, as the report's authors termed it, "forced shaving" (figure I.1). The report explained how the heads and beards of at least two of the fourteen detainees were shaved clean but for a few, irregular patches of hair, deliberately left to create an "undignified," humiliating appearance.[2] Other descriptions of detainee treatment outlined similar practices. A 2005 feature story in *Time* maga-

1

zine detailed intelligence officers' long campaign to extract information from a man named Mohammed al-Qahtani, who had been captured fleeing Tora Bora in December 2001 and sent to Guantánamo. By the fall of 2002, *Time* reported, al-Qahtani's "resilience under pressure" led officials at the detention facility to seek approval from Washington for more coercive interrogation strategies. In December of that year, then-secretary of defense Donald Rumsfeld approved more than a dozen alternative methods, including prolonged standing, extended periods of isolation, removal of clothing, and "forced grooming (shaving of facial hair etc.)."[3] According to a U.S. Department of Justice investigation, in 2002 an FBI agent similarly recommended the forced shaving of detainee Ghassan Abdullah al-Sharbi "in order to reduce his influence" among other detainees. Al-Sharbi, the agent reported, "was getting too much respect" on the cellblock for his waist-long beard; the beard was soon removed. The investigation further recorded allegations that some guards shaved off half of detainees' beards "in an effort to embarrass them," while others imposed shaving as "a punishment for detainee misconduct."[4]

In the searing debate that erupted around American treatment of detainees at Guantánamo, forced hair removal played an uncommon role. Critics of U.S. detention policies generally ignored the shaving altogether, instead focusing their condemnation on the use of waterboarding (suffocation by water).[5] In contrast, supporters of U.S. policies seized upon descriptions of beard removal as evidence that conditions at Guantánamo were, as *National Review* editor Rich Lowry put it, "nothing to be ashamed of."[6] Referring to al-Qahtani's interrogation, radio talk show host Michael Smerconish asked, "Where is the abuse? We shaved the guy's beard. We played Christina Aguilera music and we pinned 9-11 victim photos to his lapel. That's abuse?"[7] A *Washington Times* editorial, citing the *Time* magazine report, characterized the treatment of Guantánamo detainees as "unpleasant":

> [I]nterrogators did a number of unpleasant things to
> al Qahtani to get him to talk. These included shav-

ing his beard, stripping him naked, ordering him to
bark like a dog, depriving him of sleep—to the music of Christina Aguilera, no less—and violating his
"personal space" with a vulgar female interrogator.[8]

Fred Barnes, executive editor of the *Weekly Standard*, summarized the mood among the Bush administration's supporters when
he concluded that "there have been FBI reports of rough treatment [at Guantánamo], but nothing I would consider torture."[9]
Although the International Committee of the Red Cross, Human
Rights Watch, and detainees themselves repeatedly characterized
beard removal as a violation of religious belief, personal dignity,
and international treaty obligations, opponents and defenders of

Figure I.1. Table of
contents from a 2007
Red Cross report on
the treatment of U.S.-
held detainees at
Guantánamo Bay,
noting the use of
"forced shaving."

Contents

Introduction
1. Main Elements of the CIA Detention Program
   1.1. Arrest and Transfer
   1.2. Continuous Solitary Confinement
       and Incommunicado Detention
   1.3. Other Methods of Ill-treatment
       1.3.1. Suffocation by water
       1.3.2. Prolonged stress standing
       1.3.3. Beatings by use of a collar
       1.3.4. Beating and kicking
       1.3.5. Confinement in a box
       1.3.6. Prolonged nudity
       1.3.7. Sleep deprivation and use of loud music
       1.3.8. Exposure to cold temperature/cold water
       1.3.9. Prolonged use of handcuffs and shackles
       1.3.10. Threats
       1.3.11. Forced shaving
       1.3.12. Deprivation/restricted provision of solid food
   1.4. Further Elements of the Detention Regime
2. Conditions of Detention In Later Stages
3. Health Provision and Role of Medical Staff
4. Legal Aspects Related to Undisclosed Detention
5. Fate of Other Persons who Passed Through the CIA Detention Program
6. Future use of the CIA Detention Program
Conclusion
Annex 1.
Annex 2.

U.S. detention policy alike generally regarded forced shaving as a minor footnote to the nation's larger "war on terror."

The striking unity of opinion among Bush administration supporters and critics on the insignificance of forced shaving, particularly when juxtaposed with the divergent judgment of the ICRC, raises a number of questions. When exactly does a practice cease to be merely "unpleasant" and become "cruel," "inhuman" torture? What distinguishes trivial nuisances from serious problems? Who gets to determine the parameters of true suffering, and of real violence? Such questions—matters of knowledge and power, privilege and exclusion, life and death—animate this book, a history of hair removal in the United States from the colonial era to the present.

At first glance, hair removal may seem an odd subject for such rumination. The treatment of body hair, like incessant celebrity diet updates or major league sporting news, could easily be considered one of those annoying tics of contemporary American culture best ignored. The whole topic of body hair, I have learned, strikes many people as not merely tedious but also uncouth, even downright repulsive. Several previous reviewers of this work suggested that hair removal is simply too repellent to merit scholarly attention.[10]

It is not my intention to try to persuade readers otherwise. Although, as we shall see, hair removal has preoccupied political thinkers in the United States from Thomas Jefferson to Donald Rumsfeld, has shaped practices of science, medicine, commerce, and war, and has elicited breathtaking levels of financial, emotional, and ecological investment, this book does not try to argue that body hair is "in fact" more consequential than previously recognized. To do so—to assert, say, that forced shaving is actually more torturous than waterboarding—would simply flip existing presumptions of value. My aim here is instead to illuminate the historical contingency of such assertions themselves. Delving into the history of personal enhancement, *Plucked* excavates the surprisingly recent development of seemingly self-evident distinctions between the serious and the unimportant, the necessary and the superfluous.

Body hair, here referring to any hair growth below the scalp line, renders such distinctions helpfully concrete. Readily and temporarily modifiable, hair serves as a tangible medium for communicating and challenging social boundaries. The modification of hair often establishes multiple boundaries at once: not only separating self from other but also dividing and ranking "categories or classes of individuals."[11] In the United States, those classifications have long served to segregate bodies into distinct sexes, races, and species, and to delimit the numerous rights and privileges based on those distinctions. Assessments and treatments of body hair also have served to define mental instability, disease pathology, criminality, sexual deviance, and political extremism. Some classifications have been codified in diagnostic criteria, bureaucratic regulations, or technical standards; others remain tacit understandings, held fast by emotion and habit. Throughout, the maintenance of such segregations and classifications has required labor, physical and emotional labor—the often grubby, painful chore of separating hide from flesh. By examining that labor more closely, we might better perceive the implicit values suffusing social life.

OF PARTICULAR CONCERN here are ideas about suffering. In the United States, those consequential moral and legal standards— e.g., *does the treatment of detainees at Guantánamo constitute torture?*—have long been established through recourse to the "natural" order of things, as discerned by scientific and medical experts. Battles over whose suffering gets to matter have been waged, in large part, over who is authorized to speak about natural facts. In the eighteenth century, for instance, the pronouncements of bodily "deficiency" made by eminent ethnologists and naturalists helped to buttress the political disenfranchisement of the continent's indigenous peoples. In the nineteenth century, the arguments for the separate, distinct origins of races offered by physicians and anthropologists of the "American School" were summoned to defend the institution of slavery. More recently, the Behavioral Science Consultation Teams deployed at Guantánamo served to establish the parameters of "enhanced" interrogation techniques. Expert assessments of real suffering authorize specific legal procedures, and vice versa.[12]

Although definitions of suffering have been tied to claims about nature throughout U.S. history, the rising prominence of the sciences, paired with increasing emphasis on individual bodily health, amplified the significance of those scientific and medical classifications. Over the course of the nineteenth and twentieth centuries, the human body moved firmly under medicine's purview.[13] Particularly for the affluent, more and more domains of everyday life—sexuality, cognition, mood—have been moved into the province of expert assessment and treatment. Today, the boundaries of suffering—psychic and physical—are established and contested through complex, multidirectional engagements with medicine.[14]

Crucial to those boundaries are references to medical "necessity," a term that has mutated from an obscure insurance designation to the focus of national debate. Although suffering might be understood as a scalar attribute (a complaint might move up or down the ladder of "seriousness"), the concept of medical necessity acts to fence "real" suffering, allocating or withholding social and financial resources in a binary fashion.[15] Medical necessity compels for-or-against decisions. Contested diagnostic categories, such as fibromyalgia or Chronic Fatigue Syndrome, drive patient advocates as well as medical providers to seek reproducible tests of "legitimate" disease. New drugs and devices, such as memory-enhancing pharmaceuticals, demand decisions about their appropriate application. State and federal health care reforms force questions about precisely which services ought to be considered "basic" or "essential" (e.g., kidney transplants, in-vitro fertilizations, gender-reassignment surgeries). And, even as distinctions between elective "enhancement" and necessary "therapy" acquire fresh importance, accountability for the determination of these distinctions is obscured, veiled by the spread of integrated private insurance plans with capitated payment systems. As critics rightly point out, insurance companies are rarely called on to justify their exclusions.[16]

The United States is hardly exceptional in witnessing the extension of medical authority: the "biomedicalization" of everyday life has been charted across the affluent industrialized world. With time and resources, a more exhaustive comparative study—a global history of sciences of hair—would be ideal.[17] But given the disproportionate influence of U.S. definitions of "necessity" in the early twenty-first century (evident in the ICRC's report on Guantánamo), sustained reflection on American habits seems a useful place to start.

BUT FIRST, A few notes on terminology may prove helpful. Because this book seeks to emphasize the contingency of ideas often treated as timeless, I take some care to employ the terms of identity and difference used by period writers themselves (e.g., "Indian," "lunatic," "man of science"). Relying on what might be called "actors' categories" carries the obvious hazard of being misinterpreted as condoning the activities under discussion; I hope that readers will not mistake my intent in this way. To take but one example, I follow the U.S. government in using the word "detainee" to refer to the men held against their will at Guantánamo, not to convey support for indefinite detention but to stress the consequences of seemingly minute terminological decisions. "Criminals" would need to be charged with specific crimes; "prisoners" would be endowed with specific rights.[18] Elsewhere, too, I resist the impulse to simply extend idioms backwards or forwards anachronistically: the nineteenth-century "invert" is not synonymous with the twentieth-century category of "homosexual," nor "man" with "people," nor "Mongolian" with "Asian." The introduction of new words, or familiar words invested with new meaning, often signals subtle, consequential changes in thought.

I TAKE A similar approach to what might be called the "basic science" of hair and hair growth (figure I.2). Today, the terms of that science are often presented as straightforward and uncontro-

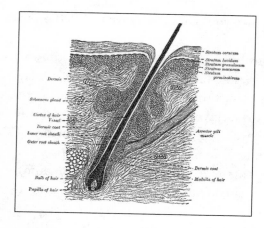

Figure I.2. Diagram of a hair follicle, from the 1918 U.S. edition of *Gray's Anatomy of the Human Body.*

versial. Mammalian hair is said to grow from follicles in the dermis (the layer of skin between the epidermis and subcutaneous tissues) into a long shaft that extends above the skin surface. The root of each hair ends in an enlargement, called the bulb, that fits like a cap over the dermal papilla. Hair fibers are further made up of three layers (medulla, cortex, and cuticle). The cortex, shaped by the follicle, helps determine the shape of the fiber and resulting texture: round fibers result in relatively straight hair, oval fibers result in relatively curly or wavy hair. Follicles also contain special stem cells, unique to the skin, that regulate the cycle of hair growth.[19] These claims, like other assertions about nature, are not arbitrary; they must respond to the material world or they will fade away. But, like all facts, they are bound to specific conditions of production—conditions that, upon closer inspection, often reveal more complexity and discord than are presented in most textbooks.[20] Take the very term "mammalian," for instance. As historian Londa Schiebinger has argued, Enlightenment taxonomists wrestled with multiple classificatory schema before landing on the category of *Mammalia*; Linnaeus chose to focus on the breast (*mammae*) rather than equally valid terms, such as *Pilosa* or *Lactentia*, in response to broader cultural and political struggles.[21] Subsequent chapters address other key scientific and medical taxonomies, including classifications of hair structure (such as distinctions between hair and feathers), type (such as Negroid or Caucasoid), and growth pattern (male or female).[22] Throughout, I refrain from placing derisive quotation marks around those words or concepts no longer seen as "scientific."

Several previous readers of this work have taken issue with this agnostic approach, asking instead for straightforward declarations of what an outdated disease category "really means," or who members of some now-defunct racial category might "actually have been" according to twenty-first-century parlance. Such requests seem to miss the point. The chief virtue of body hair as an object of historical study is that it wreaks havoc on established partitions, rendering their scaffolding unusually transparent. This book seeks to describe that scaffolding.

Many of the book's sources were produced by highly educated Anglophone writers of European descent. Many of the claims made in those sources advance specific racial, national, economic, sexual, and religious interests at the expense of others. This is not to suggest that there are no other perspectives on these matters, no alternatives to dominant attitudes and practices; again, given time and resources, a more exhaustive exploration of subcultural, subaltern, and oppositional attitudes and practices would be ideal. Here, I focus on privilege, its distortions and silences. Considered in this way, history becomes a tool of cultural critique: a way to emphasize the conflict, uncertainty, and possibility present in realms too often taken for granted.[23]

IN THE CONTEMPORARY United States, few practices are as taken for granted as the deliberate removal of body hair. (This study does not address the involuntary loss of hair associated with toxic exposures, alopecia, trichotillomania, cancer treatments, or male pattern baldness.)[24] Recent studies indicate that more than 99 percent of American women voluntarily remove hair, and more than 85 percent do so regularly, even daily. The usual targets, for the moment, are legs, underarms, eyebrows, upper lips, and bikini lines. Those habits, furthermore, appear to transcend ethnic, racial, and regional boundaries.[25] Over the course of a lifetime, one 2008 survey indicated, American women who shave (a relatively inexpensive way to remove hair) will spend, on average, more than ten thousand dollars and nearly two entire months of their lives simply managing unwanted hair. The woman who waxes once or twice a month will spend more than twenty-three thousand dollars over the course of her lifetime.[26] Most American men, too, now routinely remove facial hair, and increasing numbers modify hair elsewhere on their bodies. Research indicates that as of 2005, more than 60 percent of American men were regularly reducing or removing hair from areas of the body below the neck.[27] Although generally ignored by social scientists surveying hair removal trends, transsexual, transgender, and genderqueer people also express concern with hair management, and employ varying techniques of hair removal.[28]

The ubiquity of personal hair removal in the United States is particularly striking given its relative novelty.[29] To be clear: *forcible* hair removal is not new. The use of hair removal to control or degrade, as with the beard removals at Guantánamo, has been imposed on inmates, soldiers, students, and other captives for centuries. Despite the recent treatment of U.S. detainees, American courts have tended to frown on the forced removal of hair by agents of the state.[30] In an influential 1879 decision, U.S. Supreme Court Justice Stephen J. Field held that the San Francisco officials who cut off the long queues of Chinese men confined in county jails were in violation of both the Constitution's guarantee of equal protection and its prohibition on cruel and unusual punishment.[31] Nonstate actors also have removed hair as a way to maintain and reproduce specific relations of domination. Particularly telling in this regard were the slave traders who shaved and oiled the faces of enslaved men being prepared for sale. Because vigorous men drew higher prices, traders sometimes shaved away signs of grey beards or the first stages of pubertal growth in order to make the men appear younger. An eighteenth-century engraving of a slave market depicts an Englishman licking the face of

an enslaved man to check for telltale traces of stubble before purchase (figure I.3).[32]

Although overtly coercive hair removal has a long history in
the United States, the more widespread practices of voluntary
hair removal evident today are remarkably recent. So, too, is the
dominant culture's general aversion to visible hair.[33] From the first
decades of contact and colonization through the first half of the
nineteenth century, disdain for body hair struck most European
and Euro-American observers as decidedly peculiar: one of the
enigmatic characteristics of the continent's indigenous peoples. In
sharp contrast with the discourse surrounding bearded detainees
at Guantánamo, the beardless "Indians" were described as exceptionally, even bizarrely, eager to pluck and shave. Only in the late
nineteenth century did non-Native Americans, primarily white
women, begin to express persistent concern about their own body
hair, and not until the 1920s did large numbers begin routinely

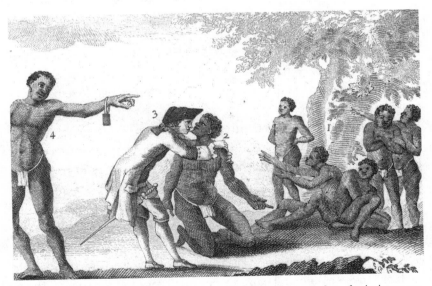

Figure I.3. An eighteenth-century engraving of a slave market, depicting a potential buyer licking an enslaved man's chin to determine whether he had been
shaved. (From *Le Commerce de l'Amerique par Marseille* [1764]. Reproduced
courtesy of the John Carter Brown Library at Brown University.)

removing hair below the neck. By the mid-twentieth century, however, the revolution was nearly complete: where eighteenth-century naturalists and explorers considered hair-free skin to be the strange obsession of indigenous peoples, Cold War–era commentators blithely described visible body hair on women as evidence of a filthy, "foreign" lack of hygiene.[34] The normalization of smooth skin in dominant U.S. culture is not even a century old.

What accounts for this increasing antipathy toward body hair? Previous historical investigation sheds little light on the matter. Even the voluminous scholarship devoted to various beauty practices in the United States—cosmetics, breast enlargements, plastic surgery, hairstyling—largely overlooks hair removal.[35] How, then, might we understand the prevalence of practices that are repetitive and expensive, at best, and not infrequently messy, painful, disfiguring, and even deadly?

SEARCHING THROUGH EXISTING scholarly and popular literatures for answers, one discovers that two broad causal stories about hairlessness turn up with special frequency: the first might be referred to as the "evolutionary" explanation, the second as the "gendered social control" explanation.[36] The sheer repetition of these two accounts is revealing. Let us therefore pause here at the outset to look at them directly.

Perhaps the most common explanation for contemporary hair removal practices, inaugurated by Desmond Morris's 1967 best-seller *The Naked Ape*, attributes the allure of hairlessness to deep, animal instinct. "Madison Avenue clearly exploits universal preferences," summarizes one recent socio-biological account, "but it does not create them."[37] Advocates of evolutionary explanations for routine hair removal often propose that the unusual hairlessness of humans—one of very few mammals to lack fur—allowed them to remain relatively free of fleas, ticks, lice, and other external parasites, along with the diseases they carry. The process of natural selection initiated by hairless hominids' greater resistance to disease was in turn augmented and reinforced by sexual selection, as potential mates responded to the unconscious messages of health and fitness conveyed through hairless skin. Contemporary *homo sapiens* allegedly maintain that ancient pattern by waxing, plucking, shaving, and so on. Another version of the theory proposes that because early bipedal hominids were under pressure to carry their infants (since bipedal infants could no longer grasp with their feet, like other primates), infant survival depended on the maternal desire to carry—a desire made stronger, so the theory goes, by the pleasure of (hairless) skin-to-skin contact. Here again, sexual selection is thought to have augmented the process of natural selection, as adults sought hairless sexual partners in order to recreate the pleasurable skin-to-skin contact of the mother-infant relationship.[38] Echoing these evolutionary lines of thought in the *Proceedings of the Royal Academy*, investigators Mark Pagel and Sir Walter Bodmer suggest that the "common use of depilatory agents testifies to the continuing attractions of hairlessness, especially in human females."[39]

The popularity of evolutionary explanations for behaviors such as the "common use of depilatory agents" points to the rising cultural authority of the sciences noted above. They also raise as many questions as they answer (as Christian creationists are quick to point out).[40] If the common use of hair removers signals the instinctual appeal of hairlessness, why would hair removal be conducted so much more diligently and obsessively in some times and places than in others? Are contemporary Americans somehow more driven by evolutionary imperative than their eighteenth-century counterparts? More than twenty-first-century Germans or Italians? If the loss of body hair provided early humans with better health and longevity, why would pubic and armpit hair remain?[41] And what's so inherently distasteful about hairy skin—to—hairy skin contact? Isn't soft, touchable fur a large part of the appeal of some domesticated animals (why they are lovingly referred to as "pets")? As one paleoanthropologist, Ian Tattersall of the American Museum of Natural History in New

York, concludes, "There are all kinds of notions as to the advantage of hair loss, but they are all just-so stories."[42]

Evolution did play a role in shaping American hair removal practices—but not because those practices reflect "Early Man's" aversion to fleas and lice.[43] Rather, the growth of evolutionary thought, particularly the influence of Charles Darwin's *Descent of Man* (1871), transformed framings of body hair, especially women's body hair. Rooted in traditions of comparative racial anatomy, evolutionary thought solidified hair's associations with "primitive" ancestry and an atavistic return to earlier, "less developed" forms. Late-nineteenth-century medical and scientific experts extended these perceptions of degeneracy, linking hairiness to sexual inversion, disease pathology, lunacy, and criminal violence. Popular culture, too, advanced hair's atavistic connotations. The display of a young, unusually hairy Laotian girl known as Krao as a "missing link," a vestigial embodiment of civilized "man's" primitive roots, exemplified this trend (figure I.4).[44] In short, readiness to attribute hair removal to the innate allure of evolutionary "fitness" is itself a consequence of cultural change.[45]

A second common explanation for Americans' intensifying pursuit of hairless skin focuses not on primordial instinct but on vested social interests: specifically, efforts to constrain women's lives. In this narrative, hair removal appears as a mechanism of "gendered social control," one exerted in proportion to women's rising economic and political power.[46] This explanation, also born of a particular historical milieu, owes much of its popularity to analyses provided by feminist social scientists. Social psychologists, in particular, have found that women who resist shaving their legs are evaluated by others as "dirty" or "gross," and that hairy women are rated as less "sexually attractive, intelligent, sociable, happy, and positive" than visibly hairless women.[47] None of this scholarship ascribes such evaluations to an orchestrated plot against women (other than the stakes that "multi-million dollar companies associated with hair removal" have in promoting the message that "hair is dirty"). Yet several studies propose that

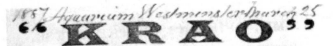

"KRAO"

THE "MISSING LINK,"

A Living Proof of Darwin's Theory of the Descent of Man.

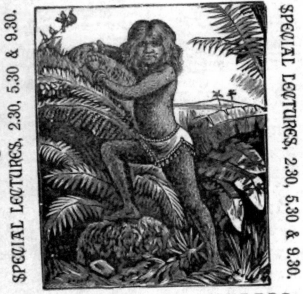

SPECIAL LECTURES, 2.30, 5.30 & 9.30.

SPECIAL LECTURES, 2.30, 5.30 & 9.30.

THE WONDER OF WONDERS.

The usual argument against the Darwinian theory, that man and monkey had a common origin, has always been that no animal has hitherto been discovered in the transmission state between monkey and man.

"KRAO,"

a perfect specimen of the step between man and monkey, discovered in Laos by that distinguished traveller, Carl Bock, will be on Exhibition in the New Lecture Room, during the Afternoon and Evening.

ALL SHOULD SEE HER.

SEE OPINIONS OF THE PRESS ON THE OTHER SIDE.

Figure I.4. An 1887 handbill presenting Krao, a young girl from Laos exhibited across the United States and Europe as a "perfect specimen of the step between man and monkey." (Courtesy of the Wellcome Library, London.)

"the hairlessness norm" imposes distinct new psychological constraints on women and girls, even as other longstanding legal and
social restrictions are eased.[48] The overall effect of the norm, social scientists suggest, is to produce feelings of inadequacy and
vulnerability, the sense that women's bodies are problematic "the
way they naturally are."[49] Practices of hair removal, in turn, are
said to produce "pre-pubescent-like," "highly sexualized" bodies,
which ultimately "may contribute to the increasing objectifica-
tion of young girls."[50]

The claim that adult hair removal is tied to the sexualiza-
tion of young women is not unfounded: some of the first fully depilated female models displayed in mass-market pornography,
such as a 1975 edition of *Hustler*, were explicitly labeled "Adolescent Fantasy."[51] It is also fair to say that the labor of maintaining
hairless skin, like many other practices of body modification in
twenty-first-century America, falls disproportionately to people
with feminine gender identities. Naomi Wolf famously referred
to the work of beautification as a "third shift" expected of women
(or, we might clarify, those who seek to be identified as women),
wedged alongside the first shift of paid work and the second shift
of unpaid household and caring work for the family.[52]

Yet the "gendered social control" narrative also suggests a
rather startling level of conformity on the part of the women being analyzed, who appear to trudge off to their repetitive, de-
meaning "third shifts" without protest. Not surprisingly, many
women balk at this depiction. Indeed, perhaps the most intriguing finding in the social-scientific literature on body hair is that
while U.S. women readily recognize the normative pressures
on them to remove their hair, and report those pressures as determining the behavior of other women, most do not accept adherence to social norms as determinative of their own practices.
Women asked to explain their own hair removal habits instead
point to increased sexual pleasure, attractiveness, and other goals
of "self-enhancement." Interviews with men establish similar
phenomena.[53] Put simply, Americans tend to describe *other* peo-

ple as dupes of social pressure, while narrating their (our) own actions as self-directed and free.

The durability of the "social control" narrative compels us to confront power-laden questions about freedom, subjectivity, and truth. Is the person who chooses to spend twenty-five hundred dollars on laser hair removal demonstrating personal liberty or a dangerous "false consciousness"? What defines false (or "true") consciousness of such choices? Who gets to say? These sorts of questions pervade contemporary discussions of breast implants, hair straightening, rhinoplasty, and other types of aesthetic "enhancement." And, as we will learn, these sorts of questions reach from the founding of the nation to the present: from eighteenth-century naturalists' arguments over whether Native men did or did not purposefully pluck their beards to more recent conflict over whether total pubic waxing constitutes personal "enslavement," American debates over body modification have entailed consternation over just how autonomous and willful apparent choices truly are.

In the end, such questions bear an important resemblance to debates over whether forced grooming at Guantánamo is "nothing to be ashamed of" or a cruel and degrading "deprivation of liberty." Common to both sets of questions is an effort to determine whether a given activity meets or exceeds some presumed standard of "freedom" or "suffering"—ignoring how those standards are set, and by whom.[54] While not indifferent to the enduring enigma of individual will, I take a different tack in this book. Rather than evaluating the choice to remove hair, I seek to show how and for whom body hair became a problem in the first place. Tracing the history of choice in this way, we see how some experiences of suffering, and not others, come to matter.

[1]

THE HAIRLESS INDIAN

Savagery and Civility before the Civil War

AMERICANS TEND TO remember Thomas Jefferson for many things, but his thoughts about hair removal are not generally among them. Nevertheless, Jefferson expressed a studied opinion on the matter in his only book, *Notes on the State of Virginia* (1785). He turned to hair in a long passage enumerating the distinctions he detected between "the Indians" and "whites":

> It has been said that the Indians have less hair than the whites, except on the head. But this is a fact of which fair proof can scarcely be had. With them it is disgraceful to be hairy on the body. They say it likens them to hogs. They therefore pluck the hair as fast as it appears. But the traders who marry their women, and prevail on them to discontinue this practice, say, that nature is the same with them as with the whites.[1]

Were Indian bodies naturally hairy like those of settlers from Europe, only appearing otherwise due to some strange habit? Or were Indian bodies irrevocably different from those of whites? Jefferson was far from the only eighteenth-century observer preoccupied with this enigma, or with the absence of "fair proof" of an answer.[2] From the 1770s through the 1850s, the enigma of

19

Native depilatory practices preoccupied European and Euro-American missionaries, traders, soldiers, and naturalists. Scores of commentators pondered whether the continent's indigenous peoples had less hair by "nature" or whether they methodically shaved, plucked, and singed themselves bare (figure 1.1).

Rarely distinguishing between the diverse indigenous peoples of the Americas in this regard (instead lumping geographically and linguistically dissimilar groups together as "Indians"), white writers both famous and now forgotten sought to explain the smooth faces and limbs that they viewed as typical of the original "Americans."[3] Cornelis de Pauw, for instance, saw the complete absence of beard as one of the distinctive physiological characteristics of Indian bodies.[4] In contrast, Meriwether Lewis and William Clark concluded that Chopunnish men "extract their beards" like "other savage nations of America," while Chopunnish women further "uniformly extract the hair below [the face]."[5] In 1814, the renowned German explorer Alexander von Humboldt conceded that even the most "celebrated naturalists" had failed to resolve whether the Americans "have naturally no beard and no hair on the rest of their bodies, or whether they pluck them carefully out."[6]

These were hardly idle musings. For European and North American observers, such questions of natural order entailed consequential questions of political order: whether Indians might be converted to European ways of life, or whether some fundamental, unalterable difference rendered assimilation impossible. The French naturalist Comte de Buffon's famous *Histoire naturelle* held to the latter position, asserting that "the peculiar environment of the New World" had "stunted" the peoples he called aborigines, making it unlikely that they could ever be "admitted to membership in the new republic."[7] As the Pennsylvania-born naturalist and traveler William Bartram posed the problem in 1791, at issue in Indian hairlessness was whether Indians might be persuaded to "adopt the European modes of civil society," or whether they were inherently "incapable of civilization" on whites' terms.[8]

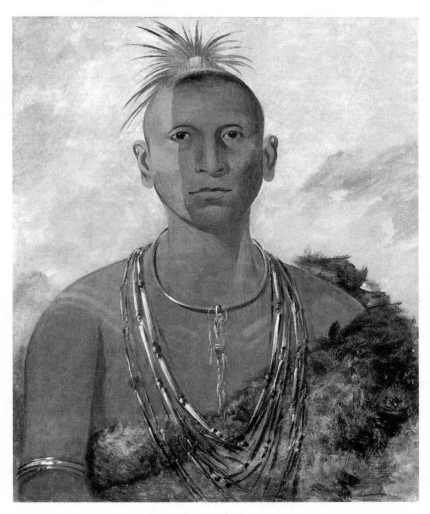

Figure 1.1. George Catlin's 1832 portrait of Náh-se-ús-kuk, eldest son of Black Hawk. Catlin, like other white travelers and naturalists of the period, was preoccupied with the smooth skin of Native peoples. (Reproduced with permission of the Smithsonian American Art Museum.)

Body hair encapsulated these debates. More than one writer claimed rights of dominance over Indian lands because, as Montesquieu explained, Native men possessed "scanty beards."[9] In this context, Jefferson himself well understood the stakes of his discussion: Native peoples' inherent rights to self-determination.[10]

With Andrew Jackson's election to the U.S. presidency in 1828, the question of Indian governance moved to the forefront of federal policy. Jackson's proposal to forcibly "remove" remaining southeastern Indians west of the Mississippi provoked fierce opposition. Nonetheless, thousands of U.S. troops were sent to Georgia, resulting in the immediate beatings, rapes, and murders of countless Cherokees, and the eventual deaths of thousands more on the Trail of Tears. By 1837, most members of the five southeastern nations had been relocated through what historian Daniel Heath Justice has characterized as a "ruthless and brutal terrorism campaign."[11] With the expansionist policies ushered in with the election of James Polk in 1844, Native peoples living in California, the Southwest, and the Northwest were subjected to similar federal jurisdiction.[12]

Whether or not white writers explicitly addressed these political developments, their perspectives on Indian body hair—the crux of debates over the nature of Indian racial character—necessarily engaged larger, ongoing disputes over the sovereignty of Native governments, the sanctity of treaties, and the appropriate use of federal force. The historical import of those disputes cannot be overstated. "If slavery is the monumental tragedy of African American experience," Tiya Miles writes, "then removal plays the same role in American Indian experience."[13] White assertions of Indian beardlessness contributed to a body of racial thought that helped to buttress those policies and practices of physical removal.[14] As the Pequot intellectual William Apess summarized in 1831, "the unfortunate aborigines of this country" have been "doubly wronged by the white man": "first, driven from their native soil by the sword of the invader, and then darkly slandered by the pen of the historian. The former has treated him like beasts of the fores[t]; the latter has written volumes to justify him in his outrages."[15]

Taken together, the volumes written about Indian body hair in the late eighteenth and early nineteenth centuries—none, so far as I have been able to locate, written by Native authors themselves—reveal the asymmetrical production of consequential standards and categories of difference. Like other "racial" differences, assessments of body hair at once reflected and supported emerging military and political regimes. But quite unlike skin color, skull size, and the myriad other anatomical characteristics used by naturalists and ethnologists to sort and rank people, body hair was both readily removable and remarkably idiosyncratic in its rate of return. Hair's unusual visibility and malleability allowed numerous, conflicting interpretations. In the midst of violent contestation over Indian policy in the eighteenth and early nineteenth centuries, those conflicting interpretations loomed large in American racial taxonomies.

It is worth emphasizing that these taxonomies are the product of European and Euro-American points of view. The few extant written accounts of Native attitudes toward hair, such as Jefferson's ("They say it likens them to hogs"), are filtered through imperial lenses. Moreover, although the writers described here often mentioned both female and male hair removal, most of the debate over Indian depilation focused on male bodies, and specifically male beards. The absence of prolonged discussion of other parts of the body—such as the female pubic region—suggests an intriguing feature of early American natural history: with regard to body hair, at least, Indian *men* were the object of naturalists' most meticulous deliberations. Given the partial nature of these accounts, they might best be approached not as conclusive descriptions of so-called Indian bodies in the eighteenth and early nineteenth centuries, but as a window into the perceptions, anxieties, and curiosities of the dominant culture. Through that window we may observe a set of questions about the nature of difference that persist to our time: What explains variation in human bodies?

How do particular environments influence the expression of heritable traits? What, in the end, is "race"?

THE USE OF hair as an index of political capacities has roots in Enlightenment natural philosophy. When Linnaeus introduced his famous system of taxonomical nomenclature in 1735, he began by asserting four distinct "varieties" of *Homo sapiens*. Hair color, type, and amount ("black, straight, thick," "yellow, brown, flowing") were the leading indicators of each variety, followed in turn by each group's alleged political characteristics, such as "regulated by customs" or "governed by caprice."[16] Buffon similarly joined body hair to capacities for reason and civility when claiming that the absence of body hair on "the American savage" reflected a deeper lack of will and motivation. The Indians' efforts represented not the deliberate exercise of reason but rather "necessary action" produced by animal impulse. "Destroy his appetite for victuals and drink," he declared, "and you will at once annihilate the active principle of all his movements."[17] The political implications of this physiological inertia were clear to Buffon: "[N]o union, no republic, no social state, can take place among the morality of their manners."[18] Hairlessness was thus thought to indicate whether indigenous peoples might be treated as equal subjects, or whether some inherent "feebleness" precluded incorporation into "civilized" modes of life.[19]

These hierarchical distinctions were themselves steeped in humoral theories dating to the classical age. Humoral theory proposed that bodies were not bounded by the envelope of the skin but were instead profoundly permeable to diet, climate, sleep, lunar movements, and other external influences. Maintaining appropriate constitutional balance among the four humors—black bile, yellow bile, phlegm, and blood—necessitated careful exchange between inside and outside, hot and cold, wet and dry. One's resulting "complexion," including body hair, was thought to reveal the balance of humors within, a balance as much moral as physiological.[20] This humoral vision was racialized as well as gendered: for European women, a pale, porcelain complexion was particularly prized; while for men, lush beard growth was thought to imply a healthy constitution. Although fashions in white men's whiskers varied across time, region, religion, occupation, and military status (Jefferson himself was generally clean-shaven, as were most U.S. presidents before Lincoln), most eighteenth-century naturalists echoed Galenic medical theory in equating thick beards with philosophical wisdom.[21]

Hence the moral and physiological question, Was the Indian's seemingly smooth skin similarly subject to external influence? If so, which influences, exactly? Given the weighty political implications of their conclusions, European and Euro-American writers energetically debated the extent to which Indian complexion might be affected by food, weather, and mode of life. In a 1777 book used as a standard reference on Indians in both Europe and the United States until well into the nineteenth century, Scottish historian William Robertson concluded that the answer was no: the hairless skin of the Americans instead provided evidence of "natural debility."[22] "They have no beard," he wrote in his *History of the Discovery and Settlement of North America*, "and every part of their body is perfectly smooth," a "feebleness of constitution" mirrored in their aversion to "labour" and their incapacity for "toil."[23] Robertson insisted that the "defect of vigour" indicated by the Indian's "beardless countenance" stemmed not from rough diet or harsh environment but from an inherent "vice in his frame."[24] Although "rude tribes in other parts of the earth" subsist on equally simple fare, he maintained, Indians alone remained "destitute of [this] sign of manhood."[25]

Robertson was challenged on exactly that point by Samuel Stanhope Smith, later president of Princeton University. In the influential *Essay on the Causes of the Variety of Complexion and Figure in the Human Species*, Smith argued that apparent differences between white and Indian bodies were overblown. "The celebrated Dr. Robertson," Smith chided in 1787, joined "hasty, ignorant observers" in claiming that "the natives of America

have no hair on the face, or the body," thus binding him "to account for a fact which does not exist." Although "careless travelers" saw a "deficiency" of hair and presumed a "natural debility
of constitution," Indians were no different "from the rest of the
human race" in this regard. As Smith concluded, the "hair of
our native Indians, where it is not carefully extirpated by art,
is both thick and long."[26] In Smith's perspective, the "common
European error" that "the natives of America are destitute of
hair on the chin, and body" was vile not simply because it revealed a striking observational ineptness but more importantly
because it ran counter to Genesis. Smith stressed the influence
of diet, grooming, and other habits on perceived differences in
hair growth as a way to affirm scriptural teachings on the unity
of creation.[27]

As Smith's essay on the causes of human variety suggests, lurking in descriptions of hair removal was a pressing concern: whether
purposeful activity might effect lasting changes to physical form.
From where did apparent differences between races, sexes, or species arise, if not from separate creations? The great German natural philosopher Johann Blumenbach, for instance, proposed that
the "scanty" hair typical of "Americans" could indeed result from
daily grooming. Repeated "mutilations" such as "extirpat[ing] the
beard" and "eradicating the hair in different parts of the body," he
claimed, could result in more permanent differences in form.[28] For
Blumenbach, Indian hair removal exemplified how human variation might be "occasioned by . . . artificial means."[29] The English
naturalist James Cowles Prichard flatly rejected this perspective.
Declaring variation in the "quantity of hair that grows on the human body" (particularly the "deficiency" of hair "ascribed to all
the American nations") to be one of the "well-known differences
between races," Prichard scoffed at the idea that such persistent
differences might be acquired by plucking and shaving.[30] Where
Blumenbach and others "conjectured that the habit of pulling out
the hair through many generations" may produce distinct varieties
of people, hairlessness was far too general a trait "to be ascribed to

so accidental a cause."[31] Instead, in a passage that augured Darwin's controversial theory of sexual selection, Prichard argued that an "instinctive perception of human beauty . . . implanted by Providence" helped "direct" men in their marriages, ultimately shaping the divergent appearances of the human form. This providential love of beauty (which Prichard assumed to favor denuded skin) acts "as a constant principle of improvement," akin to man's selective breeding of particularly fine animal specimens. Prichard thus explained the relative hairlessness of humans through reference to a divinely implanted aesthetic preference.[32] Prichard offered no indication of how Providence might account for the fact, as Blumenbach put it, that some parts of the human body, such as the armpit or groin, were evidently "more hairy than in brute animals," or the equally confounding idea that Europeans might be hairier than Indians.[33] Smooth, hairless skin presented a conundrum in this regard, as it was at once one of the distinguishing characteristics of "the Indian" and also, in Blumenbach's terms, one of the chief "diagnostic signs by which man differs from other mammals."[34] Such distinctions had to come from somewhere.

THE IDEA THAT perceived distinctions between peoples could be shaped by deliberate effort—that racial characteristics might be cultivated and transmitted—dominated U.S. Indian policy in the first decades of the republic. As Henry Knox, the nation's first secretary of war, argued to Congress in 1789, while "it has been conceived to be impracticable to civilize the Indians of North America," evidence of Indian improvement is clear from "the progress of society, from the barbarous ages to its present state of perfection."[35] Belief that Indians could "progress" from savagery through barbarism to civilization shaped early federal policy—even as that policy bobbed between treating Native men as capable of entering legal agreements and treating them as requiring paternalistic protection.[36]

But by 1819, white settlers in the young republic had largely filled the tens of millions of acres already seized from Native peoples. Public pressure for cession of additional land grew accordingly.[37] Resistance to white colonization was met with claims that Indians were "intellectually and morally incapable of forming true governments," and investigations of the inherent "deficiencies" of Indian bodies came to the fore.[38] Increasingly in agreement that Indians *were* less hairy than whites, white observers focused their debate on whether the relative hairlessness of Indians resulted from "careful extirpation," as Smith would have it, or some more "imperishable" anatomical trait.[39]

Observers remained divided, for example, over whether Indian men were able to permanently end beard growth by repeatedly extracting it at the onset of puberty. In his 1841 account of travels into Native American territory, George Catlin declared that among tribes that made no efforts to imitate whites, most men "by nature are entirely without the appearance of a beard." Of those with some beard growth, "nineteen out of twenty" eradicated it permanently by "plucking it out several times in succession, precisely at the age of puberty."[40] Others joined Catlin in proposing that Indians were able to "arrest" the involuntary growth of hair at puberty through deliberate labor.[41] The Slovenian missionary Frederic Baraga disputed accounts that portrayed the "Indians as a naturally beardless people," and asserted that Indian hair growth ceases because "young men take the greatest care to pull out or burn the first fuzz which covers their chins."[42] Eugene Blandel, a young soldier with the westward-pushing U.S. Army, conveyed a similar idea in an 1856 letter to his family: "[N]one of these Indians wears a beard. All hair on the face is pulled out by the roots, as soon as it makes its appearance, so that it never grows again."[43]

Whites' preoccupation with the nature of Indian bodies also pervaded their descriptions of which tools, if any, Indians used to remove their hair. The Natchez of the lower Mississippi were said to pluck with clamshells or copper tweezers, the Sanpoil of Eastern Washington to use bone or wooden tweezers, and the Assiniboine to use "small wire tweezers of their own make."[44] The

Pennsylvania natural historian Samuel Stehman Haldeman conveyed an account of an indigenous woman shaving a child's head with a "shark's tooth fastened to the end of a stick" and of men shaving with two shells—"one being placed under some of the beard, the other used to cut or scrape above."[45] Members of the Iroquois Confederacy were said to have special instruments "for the purpose of plucking," save for "a very small number, who, from living among white people, have adopted their customs." Iroquois who live with whites, one military surgeon noted, "sometimes have razors."[46] Exasperated with the repeated claim that "the Indians are beardless by nature and have no hair on their bodies," in 1818 the Reverend John Heckewelder declared that the idea should be "exploded and entirely laid aside." "I cannot conceive how it is possible for any person to pass three weeks only among those people," he snorted, "without seeing them pluck out their beards, with tweezers made expressly for that purpose" from sharpened mussel shells or brass wire. These tweezers "they always carry with them in their tobacco-pouch, wherever they go, and when at leisure, they pluck out their beards or hair above their foreheads," with quick strokes "much like the plucking of a fowl." The "oftener they pluck out the hair, the finer it grows afterwards, so that at last there appears hardly any, the whole having been rooted out."[47] The most remarkable aspect of Indian hairlessness, other observers concurred, was that Indian men and women so methodically and ceaselessly removed their body hair, which they viewed as a "deformity" or "vulgarity."[48]

The emphasis on continual, painstaking cultivation of the body evident in these accounts is noteworthy, given that whites generally depicted Indians as particularly *averse* to labor. (Recall Buffon's insistence that Indian activities were limited to those directed by bestial appetites, or Robertson's condemnation of Indians' constitutional torpor.)[49] With respect to body hair, though, the Indian was said to be exceedingly diligent, ready to subject his chin to the "repeated pains" of extractions "nearly every day of his life."[50] The Indian's alleged willingness to suffer in this

regard was a point of ethnographic fascination, even consternation, as Jefferson emphasized in his remarks on white traders' Indian wives. Surely no "civilized" person would be so peculiarly
invested in plucking, shaving, and singeing.

ATTENTION TO THE "mutilations" of Indian hair removal began
to wane as Indian assimilation and resistance moved to the margins of national political discussion. Responsibility for Indian
affairs was transferred from the War Department to the new Department of the Interior in 1849, and most whites slowly ceased
regarding the status of the continent's indigenous peoples as a significant military concern.[51] Preoccupation with Indian beards appears to have receded accordingly. Although the enigma of Indian
hair removal continued to surface from time to time—as late as
1849, French traveler Ernest De Massey wrote of the beardless
peoples he encountered in California, "I cannot say whether this
is natural or the result of some method of hair-removal"[52]—by
midcentury the locus of political attention had shifted to southern slavery and an emerging industrial order.[53]

Yet even as whites' fascination with Indian hair removal receded, comparative studies of body hair, brought to the fore by
Indian removal, remained a central tool of racial classification.
With the ascendance of a distinctly "American school" of ethnology in the 1830s and 1840s, comparative assessments of hair
proliferated. Dedicated to the proposition that different races derived from multiple, distinct origins, American-school ethnologists stressed the methodological rigor that they brought to their
taxonomies. Recognizing the threat that their work posed to Genesis, ethnologists like Josiah Clark Nott, George R. Gliddon, and
Samuel George Morton sought to counter arguments for a single
creation with the "patient examination of facts." Detailed measurement of hair shape, texture, and amount featured promi-
nently in these efforts. Microscopic evaluations of hair were said
to reveal fundamental distinctions between races and fundamental similarities between so-called lower races and other animals.

These claims then were used to support the continuing enslavement of men, women, and children of African descent.[54]

One of the most influential of these ethnologists, the Philadelphia microscopist and lawyer Peter A. Browne, applied his various physiological classifications of "pile" to a variety of disputes in the mid-nineteenth century: legal questions of individual racial character, medical classifications of lunacy, and ethnological debates over the "origin of the aborigines of America."[55] In one well-circulated 1853 treatise, Browne endorsed the continuation of slavery

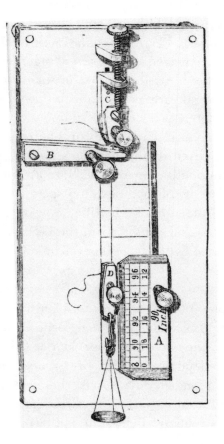

Figure 1.2. The "trichometer" developed by Peter A. Browne to assess typological differences in hair. (From *Trichologia Mammalium* [1853].)

on the basis of his discernment of "three distinct species of human beings" characterized by hair type. Citing Jefferson's earlier comparisons of "whites" and "Indians" to buttress his claims, Browne selected samples of each of those types—cylindrical ("a full-blood Choctaw Indian"), oval ("his Excellency General George Washington"), and eccentrically elliptical ("a pure Negro")—and examined them with new tools designed to measure and compare hair: the trichometer, the discotome, and the hair revolver.[56] In another widely reprinted lecture, Browne offered his examination of differences in "national pile" as a complement to Morton's famous studies of skulls, Samuel Haldeman's studies of the organs of speech, and Marie-Jean-Pierre Flourens's studies of skin color—all of them "sister sciences" dedicated to understanding the natural history of "man."[57] (Morton himself, architect of American racial taxonomies, devoted several early pages of his influential *Crania Americana* to racial differences in hair type, number, and color.)[58]

This zeal for counting and analyzing hairs as a way to establish difference continued for generations, gaining strength alongside the institutionalization of the "human sciences." Indeed, hierarchical concepts of race, sex, and species were given fresh heft by the consolidation of scientific organizations, professions, and agencies.[59] One such institution, the U.S. Sanitary Commission, was organized by the federal government after the outbreak of the Civil War. The commission's primary objective was to maintain the vitality of Union troops. Recognizing the unusual opportunities presented by the vast number of volunteer soldiers, the commission also conducted a large-scale anthropometric survey of Union recruits. Commissioner Charles J. Stillé boasted that the results of the study would "afford the most important contribution of observations ever made in furtherance of 'anthropology,' or the science of man."[60] In 1864, the well-known Boston mathematician and astronomer Benjamin Apthorp Gould was tasked with systematizing the gargantuan collection of physical data, completing the statistical calculations, and publishing the eventual findings.[61] In the resulting 613-page report, Gould took up the question, sparked by Peter Browne's earlier studies, of "the relative amount of pilosity, or general hairiness of the body."[62]

As ever, establishing evidence of such intimate matters proved a challenge. Where Thomas Jefferson based his findings about hair on the reports of white traders involved with Indian women, Gould asked an officer deployed with the 25th Army Corps on the Texan border to "avail himself of any opportunity . . . to observe the colored troops when unclothed." Observations were to be recorded according to a standard scale: "[S]kin apparently smooth should be denoted by 0, and an amount of general hairiness equal to the maximum which he had ever seen or should see in a white man, should be called a 10." The officer fulfilled the request expediently by "observing the men while bathing, which was an event of almost daily occurrence in the torrid climate near the mouth of the Rio Grande."[63] On the basis of the officer's figures, collected from more than twenty-one hundred soldiers, Gould concluded that there was "little, if any, difference between the white and black races" with respect to body hair.[64]

Gould's massive study, spawned by earlier anatomical classifications of hair, informed most American sciences of race in the second half of the nineteenth century.[65] Moreover, his observations, along with the earlier studies of George Catlin, would soon provide the evidence for Charles Darwin's controversial theories—with lasting consequences for subsequent ideas about race, sex, and hair.

[2]

"CHEMICALS OF THE TOILETTE"

From Homemade Remedies
to a New Industrial Order

ALTHOUGH TRAVELERS AND naturalists' fascination with Indian plucking and shaving would seem to indicate that whites themselves possessed no analogous habits, the prevalence of recipes for homemade hair removers in eighteenth-century domestic manuals and etiquette guides suggests that some of their contemporaries, at least, were seasoned hands at hair removal. Steeped in the same humoral theories of health that informed the work of Linnaeus, Buffon, and other prominent natural philosophers, ordinary colonial women viewed facial complexion as a reflection of underlying temperament and spirit. An "unblemished" face was a primary standard of physical beauty in the eighteenth century, an achievement distinguished, in part, by upper lips and temples free of visible fuzz. The woman afflicted by a troublingly "low forehead" might find an array of recipes for homemade pastes and powders to alleviate the problem.[1]

In the first decades of the nineteenth century, however, these time-worn domestic remedies began to be replaced by packaged commodities, which drew hair removal into emerging, opaque systems of manufacturing in novel ways. As long as economic development remained centered in the individual household or plantation and its surrounding farmland, women maintained crucial positions in the production of food, fabric, candles, medicines, and other household goods. Tools for hair removal, too, were created within

35

the household, concocted primarily by women and girls for their own use—or, in the case of enslaved and indentured women, for the use of other women in the household. But as the uneven process of industrial development unfolded, women gradually were less and less likely to weave their own cloth, preserve their own meat, or mold their own soap. Similarly, women and girls who sought to clear their complexions of hair became less likely to make their own depilatory compounds than to purchase them premade, relying as they did so on industrial-grade chemicals of unknown, often dubious quality. That reliance gave rise to understandable ambivalence about whether potentially injurious commercial hair removers might cause more suffering than the "disfiguring" growths they were meant to remedy—a concern reflected and assuaged in the marketing of the new commodities as based on ancient "Eastern" or "Oriental" beauty recipes.

THE PALE, UNBLEMISHED face so central to eighteenth-century European standards of feminine beauty was no less valued in early-nineteenth-century America. Like scars or red blotches, visible hairs on the face or neck—those areas of the female body exposed by prevailing modes of dress—were considered "deformities" anathema to the reigning porcelain ideal.[2] Physiognomy, the study of physical appearance revived and popularized most effectively by the Swiss clergyman Johann Kaspar Lavater, picked up on humoralism's emphasis on complexion as a reflection of inner character. Lavater and his followers similarly correlated the distinctive pallor of racially and economically privileged women with moral virtue, valorizing the pale, smooth feminine face with the authority of physiognomic expertise.[3]

Despite the moral stigma associated with a faint moustache or troublingly "low forehead," antebellum women suffering from conspicuous hair had few good options at their disposal. Sticky plasters made from shoemakers' waxes or tree resins were available, but appear to have been used primarily in the treatment of ringworm and other ailments.[4] Most nonenslaved women probably avoided shaving their faces for the same reason that so many men did: in the eighteenth and early nineteenth centuries, shaving could be an unpleasant, even dangerous experience. Most shaving was accomplished with a sharpened edge of metal known as a "free hand" or "cut throat" razor, the use of which required both careful maintenance and considerable skill. As one scholar of shaving summarizes, "bloodbaths could only be prevented by experienced hands."[5] Sporadic reports of syphilis being transmitted by unskilled barbers—possible through direct contact with open sores—may have increased reluctance to shave.[6] Prior to the advent of covered "safety" razors at the turn of the twentieth century, shaving was a relatively rarefied activity: men of means did not shave themselves, but instead relied on the services of skilled barbers.[7]

Barbering itself, moreover, was a craft dominated by men. In colonial America, as in eighteenth-century England, barbering was associated with bone setting, tooth extraction, bloodletting (to rebalance humors), and other aspects of medical "physick." Until 1745, barbers shared a guild with surgeons, as fellow craftsmen engaged in the manual manipulation of bodies. Surgeons eventually severed their historic ties with barber-surgeons to create a distinct medical specialty, one more closely aligned with physicians and their learned, gentlemanly rank. Even then, women remained excluded from the skilled occupation of barbering just as they were from the medical professions. In multiple ways, then, antebellum American women were discouraged from using or submitting their faces and necks to the blade.[8]

Homemade depilatories therefore offered an appealing and relatively accessible alternative for banishing visible hair. In the context of a general aversion for "face-painting" in the eighteenth and nineteenth centuries (powder and rouge were negatively associated with both aristocracy and prostitution), depilatories fell into the category of efforts to "transform the skin" that were considered generally socially acceptable. From the first years of white settlement in the New World through the turn of the nineteenth century, recipes for homemade depilatories were widespread, found throughout period cookery and etiquette manuals and passed from family member to family member and from neighbor to neighbor along with other domestic knowledge.[9]

A typical depilatory recipe appears in one of the most important English-language books on midwifery, *The Byrth of Mankynde*. First published in 1540, the book was reprinted numerous times over the subsequent century, influencing popular medicine across the American colonies. Along with other medical and domestic remedies, this "Woman's Book" offered a detailed recipe for a homemade hair remover. "TO TAKE HAYRE FROM PLACES WHERE IT IS UNSEEMLY," the recipe explained,

> Take new burnt Lime foure ounces, of Arseneck an ounce, steepe both these in a pint of water the space of two days, and then boyle it in a pint to a half. And to prove whether it be perfect, dippe a feather therein, and if the plume of the feather depart off easily, then it is strong enough: with this water then anoint so farre the place yee would have bare from hayre, as it liketh you, and within a quarter of an houre pluck at the hayres and they will follow, and then wash that place much with water wherein Bran hath been steeped: and that done, anoint the place with the white of a new laid Egge and oyle Olive, beaten and mixt together with the juyce of Singrene or Purflaine, to allay the heat engendred of the foresaid lee.[10]

If women followed these elaborate instructions, those whose "hayre groweth so low in the foreheads and the temples, that it disfigureth them" might be saved.[11] Such colonial depilatory recipes were as varied as they were complex. One influential sixteenth-century formula suggested boiling liquor calcis (a lime solution), silver paint, and aromatic oil together, soaking a rag in the result-

ing compound, and applying it to the hairy skin.[12] A single seventeenth-century manual, Johann Jacob Wecker's widely circulated
book, *Cosmeticks; or, The Beautifying Part of Physick*, contained
more than three-dozen recipes for ointments to hinder or remove
hair.[13] Others proposed applications of eggshells, vinegar, and cat's
dung, or thinning the eyebrows with a combination of ground ivy,
gum, ant eggs, burnt leeches, and frog's blood.[14]

These depilatories, part of larger traditions of folk medicine,
merged English, French, and Spanish practices with Native
American and African pharmacopeias in technically complicated
ways.[15] Although generally based on relatively simple raw materials such as spurge or acacia, hair-removing concoctions required
considerable judgment and skill in their preparation, as suggested
by the lengthy description in *The Byrth of Mankinde*.[16] Some ingredients were highly combustible; others could lead to severe
skin irritation or systemic poisoning for those who handled them
carelessly.[17] Like the production of homemade abortifacients, medicinal tinctures, and the countless other items produced in early
American households, creating effective preparations for hair removal relied on considerable hands-on knowledge and skill.[18]

INDUSTRIAL CHANGE ERODED that expertise. To be sure, the shift
from household to industrial production did not unfold along a
single, uniform trajectory. Industrial change occurred piecemeal,
varying from product to product and from nation to nation.[19]
Even solely within the United States, early industry took many
forms. Some enterprises relied on water-powered machines, others on manual labor. Some focused on highly trained artisanal
work, others on unskilled, specialized tasks. Some developed factories with dozens of employees; others remained in small shops.
Some depended on enslaved workers, others on contract laborers
supervised by managers. Some were financed by distant stock-
holders, others by capital from their on-site owners.[20]

The production of depilatories reflected these uneven developments, as individual households, particularly those in New

England and the mid-Atlantic, moved stutteringly into the exchange of goods produced by strangers. Yet where many other aspects of women's domestic labor, such as cooking and cleaning, were mechanized late in the century or not at all, homemade depilatories already were facing pressure from prefabricated alternatives by the turn of the nineteenth century.[21] Advertisements for ready-made powders and creams to "take off all superfluous hair" began appearing in U.S. newspapers and magazines as early as 1801; packaged depilatories were available to women in European towns and cities even earlier.[22] Marketed primarily though not exclusively to women, the powders promised to alleviate "unsightly appendages" from upper lips, foreheads, temples, and brows. The white face, still thought to mirror inner moral and spiritual qualities, remained the focus of commercial attention.[23]

While the precise composition of such products is unclear (and likely varied enormously from batch to batch when first produced), most would have worked in largely the same way: chemically softening or dissolving the hair so that it could be readily scraped or wiped from the surface of the skin. Some compositions, such as thallium compounds, produced a systemic toxicity that resulted in hair loss as well as nerve damage or death; arsenic compounds could produce vomiting, convulsions, coma, and death as well as hair loss. Twenty-first-century biochemists might explain that most depilatory compounds hydrolyze the disulfide bonds of keratin, the fibrous protein that makes up hair. Keratin's sulfur-to-sulfur bonds, they would say, make hair strong and flexible; when those bonds are broken chemically, hair becomes weak and pliable enough to be wiped off with a cloth or putty knife, leaving the follicle intact. Makers of early depilatories, however, had no conception of disulfide bonds or hydrolyzing action. Depilatories predate the very word "keratin," which the *Oxford English Dictionary* traces to an 1847 anatomical encyclopedia.[24]

Although the precise chemical composition of the various hair removers was obscure even to producers, interest in such packaged depilatories grew rapidly, alongside urban markets. Over the first half of the nineteenth century, dozens of small manufacturers began to concoct special blends of hair removing powders or unguents, marketed under signature labels: Trent's Depilatory, Hubert's Roseate Powder, Dr. Gouraud's Poudres Subtile. Colley's Depilatory was said to entail a mixture of "quicklime and sulphuret of potass." Devereux's Depilatory Powder could be purchased wholesale in New York City. Dillingham and Bicknell offered a "Chinese Hair Eradicator and Depilatory Powder" to shoppers in Augusta, Maine.

The sale of these goods, like that of other patent remedies, established networks of marketing and distribution later followed by manufacturers of soaps, cigarettes, and other commodities.[25] In the antebellum period, the word "patent" was used to refer to any preparation whose availability was extended through advertising—whether or not it possessed an actual government patent. Patent hair removers were distributed through wholesalers like druggists (who ordered in bulk and redistributed material to middle men) and through the apothecaries, physicians, barbers, and perfumers who sold goods directly to users.[26] Antebellum circulars, catalogues, and advertisements indicate that numerous manufacturers of patent depilatories delivered their products to consumers through a variety of strategies. One crucial factor in the development of national markets in such commodities was their relative transportability, historian James Harvey Young has shown, as shipping costs for patent medicines represented a smaller proportion of their total price than of heavier, bulkier commodities.[27] Even before the development of the transnational highways and railways that expedited industrial growth, lightweight powders and pastes could be hauled by riverboat or railroad, by foot or horse-drawn wagon. Competing fiercely with one another, larger companies might have a dozen or more distributors on the road at one time, each covering a particular district. Such efforts appear to have been successful; by the end of the Civil War, few domestic manuals contained recipes for homemade depilatories. Those troubled by facial hair would turn instead to packaged compounds such as Trent's, Devereux's, and Gouraud's.[28]

Although impossible to quantify precisely, it is clear that markets in commercial depilatories never approached the scale of markets in, say, manufactured textiles, milled flour, or boots and shoes. In 1849, for instance, the value of *all* domestic toiletry manufactures (including but not limited to depilatories) came to about $355,000, while by 1850 cotton and woolen textile production totaled more than $65 million. Certainly the role played by commercial depilatories in directing the course of industrial manufacturing should not be overstated. Yet neither should these commodities' influence on the course of American industry be underestimated. It is worth recalling that small-scale artisanal manufactories of the sort that produced depilatories remained the dominant mode of commodity production through the 1830s and 1840s. Even in Britain, the average textile factory employed fewer than one hundred people.[29] The increasing popularity of packaged hair removers in the 1810s and 1820s, like the gradual, uneven transfer of cloth production from the household treadle looms to the water-powered factories dotting the rivers of New England, signaled an emerging reliance on manufactured goods—one made possible through the application of new chemical and mechanical arts.

One of the leading products of the age, Atkinson's depilatory, exemplifies these new goods.[30] Developed by an entrepreneur who billed himself as the "perfumer to the [British] Royal Family," Atkinson's was a mixture of one part ground orpiment (a common sulfide mineral), six parts quicklime, and a little flour.[31] Generally applied to the face and neck, it was designed to remove "superfluous" hair, which advertisements routinely described as the greatest "blemish" a woman might possess. "This great disfigurement of female beauty," one advertisement in the *Liberator* explained, "is effectually removed by this article, which is perfectly safe, and easily applied, and certain in its effects" (figure 2.1).[32] Although appearing in newspapers with both black and white readers, Atkinson's advertisements presumed that pale, hairless complexion was desired: one advertisement noted that the product would not merely remove "superfluous Hair" but also leave "the skin soft and whiter than before the application."[33]

Atkinson's was also representative in another way: the manufacturers of packaged depilatories appear to have been mostly men, despite women's longstanding proficiency with home-made hair removers. This fact is remarkable: more generally, the manufacture of cosmetics in early-nineteenth-century America provided uncommon opportunities for women entrepreneurs, prospects unavailable in more guild-oriented, male-dominated occupations such as hairdressing, wig making, and barbering.[34] By the second half of the nineteenth century, some women entrepreneurs were moving to the forefront of American cosmetics production, including Ellen Demorest (born in 1824), Madam C. J. Walker (1867), Helena Rubenstein (1870), and Elizabeth Arden (1884).[35] Little evidence suggests, however, that women were similarly involved in the production or marketing of the packaged depilatories circulating in antebellum America.[36]

The relative paucity of women making and selling packaged depilatories points to the products' unusual position at the conflu-

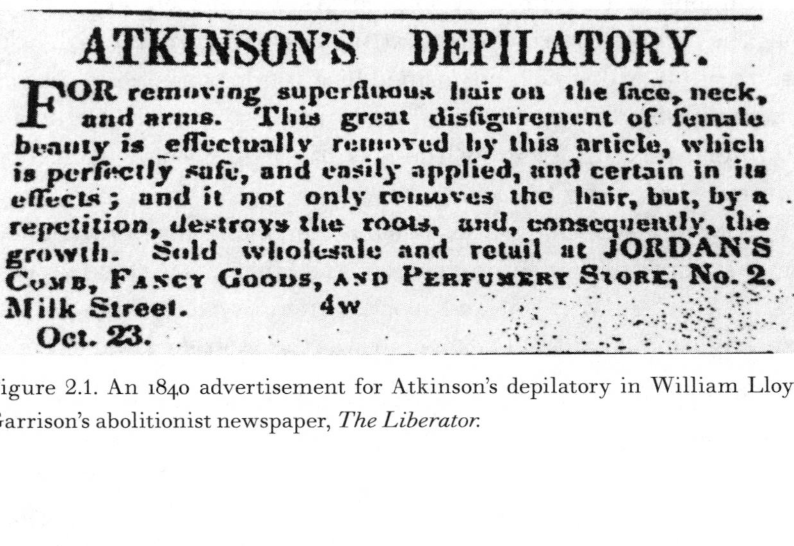

Figure 2.1. An 1840 advertisement for Atkinson's depilatory in William Lloyd Garrison's abolitionist newspaper, *The Liberator*.

ence of folk medicine and newly centralized meat production—a domain of industry heavily dominated by men. Throughout the eighteenth century, when city dwellers accounted for only a small fraction of the nation's population, most Americans reared and slaughtered their own animals. In the first federal census of 1790, there were only twenty-four cities in the country, and only two of those cities had populations exceeding 25,000. By 1840, however, the percentage of Americans living in cities had more than doubled, the number of cities had jumped to 131, and the population of New York City alone exceeded 250,000.[37] As settlements expanded and became too crowded for individuals or families to rear their own livestock, centralized stockyards and slaughterhouses grew accordingly, further segregating humans from other domesticated animals.

The expansion of centralized meat production spawned new investment in hair removal. Killing itself was not the tricky part of mass meat production; prior to the advent of mechanized refrigeration, the more complicated issue was distributing the meat as quickly as possible once the animal was dead. Focus thus turned to the problem of securing efficient, uninterrupted dismemberment. A giant moving chain, from which dead pigs were hung, conveyed the highly perishable animal through a "disassembly" line—credited by Henry Ford as an inspiration for his continuous factory production line. As with automobile assembly, the complex work of dismantling a large animal was divided into minute tasks, each performed by a single worker: repetitively chopping, breaking, stripping, packing. To the goal of efficient, uninterrupted disassembly, the task of stripping hair from hides presented a vexing bottleneck.[38]

Prior to the mechanization of slaughter, individual animal hides were stripped of hair through a gory and laborious manual process. Skins, covered with soil and blood, generally would be scrubbed clean of residual animal flesh. Hair was then softened and loosened by soaking the skin in urine, lime, or salt, and then scraped clean—

"scudded"—by hand. To complete the transition from rawhide to imperishable leather, the skin would be pounded and kneaded, often with dung used as an emollient, and then stretched and dried.[39] Foul-smelling from the combination of urine, feces, and decomposing flesh, these tanning operations were generally confined to the outskirts of town near moving water where waste could be dumped. With the increase in animal processing made possible by systematic disassembly, industrialists experimented with faster, less labor-intensive techniques of "unhairing" (figure 2.2). Scores of inventors sought new methods for expediting the process of transforming a living animal to its exchangeable and constitutive parts. As with the introduction of overhead conveyer chains in the disassembly process, experimenters sought to substitute nonhuman labor for human manual work.[40]

Where hair was concerned, many of the most effective labor-saving arts turned out to be chemical, as the influential industrial philosopher Andrew Ure noted in his widely read dictionary of mechanical arts.[41] Adapting techniques of hair removal reaching back centuries, inventors scaled up the conversion of hairy living animals into meat, leather, and wool, deepening knowledge of industrial chemistry in the process. Alkalis such as lime (calcium hydroxide) and soda ash (sodium carbonate) were most common, but various combinations of sulfides, cyanides, and amines were also developed to help weaken and strip hair.[42] Public waters became a convenient receptacle for chemically pulped hair, with damaging results. The degraded hair released noxious ammonia odors, a stench intensified by the sulfides used in unhairing. Because loose hair and caked lime tended to coat pipes and clog drainages, the effect on waterways was magnified.[43] Although toxic, the success of the novel chemical techniques was palpable: by 1830, according to one agricultural journal, the domestic manufacture of hides and skin was worth at least $30 million per year—more than $3.5 million more than total cotton exports from the United States.[44]

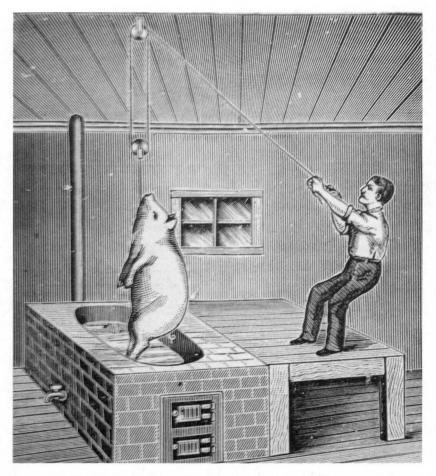

Figure 2.2. Dehiding pigs by scalding. The rise of mass meat production prodded innovation in chemical hair removal. (From *Douglas's Encyclopedia* [1902].)

EXISTING SOURCES DO not reveal the precise scope or direction of influence among what might now be considered "cosmetic," "medical," and "agricultural" applications of these industrial chemicals. Whether innovations in beautification drove agricultural applications or the other way around remains uncertain. What is clear is that the same technical knowledge that advanced mass animal processing circulated among antebellum toiletry manufacturers: compounds found to help remove hair from hogs might also strip hair from "the human skin," as Andrew Ure put it, and vice versa.[45] One representative technical manual, *The Art of Perfumery*, proposed that the same chemical depilatory designed for "ladies" who consider hair on the upper lip "detrimental to beauty" would work equally well for "tanners and fellmongers" preparing hides and skins.[46]

Quite unlike the bovine and porcine hair removal conducted in large, centralized abattoirs, however, human depilatory use was geographically dispersed. Antebellum women's hair removal remained confined to the isolation of the private home or physician's office, where the noxious smells of sulfide and ammonia and the mess of pulped hair were generally hidden from the wider public. Visible injuries resulting from the use of caustic depilatories, on the other hand, were not so easily veiled. As a result, concern about changing arts of human hair removal focused not on noxious odors or water contamination but on their more immediate risk to the complexion.[47]

Numerous commentators worried that solvents "energetic" enough to penetrate and destroy the roots of hair could also be dangerous to women's skin. (Fellmongers had related worries, as "injurious" chemical depilatories threatened to reduce the commercial value of hides.)[48] The safety of packaged depilatories— malodorous and irritating at best, lethal at worst—became a persistent concern in antebellum publications. Particularly as commercial preparations began to range beyond familiar household ingredients to include industrially produced chemicals, purchasers became increasingly unsure about just what they might be putting on their faces.[49] Occasionally, the potential for injury from packaged depilatories was treated as a source of humor. In 1804, one Boston weekly reported the "amusing" case of a "dowager lady" who followed an advertisement for a *"depilatory,* or some such name." The woman rubbed the product around her mouth, removing the hairs yet "taking all the flesh with them." Because the product "affected her eyes too" (again, some depilatory ingredients could have systemic effects), the injury "obliged her, for some time, to use a black shade; which, with her large mouth, made her look for all the world like Harlequin in a pantomime."[50]

Other descriptions did not poke fun at the new dangers facing women. The popular *Saturday Evening Post* printed a recipe for an "Oriental *rusma*," a depilatory made from quicklime, along with a warning to readers that the "very powerful" paste should be used only "with great circumspection." (The arsenic included in this particular recipe compounded the risk.)[51] An 1831 article in *Lady's Book* described packaged depilatories comprised of "a preparation of quicklime, or of some other alkaline or corrosive substance." Such corrosives, the article warned, often result in "very considerable" injuries to the skin, sores that may be "still more unsightly than the defect they were employed to remedy." Arsenic-based compounds, in particular, pose "the utmost risk to health, if not to life." The article repeated a conclusion presented in the *Journal of Health* earlier that year: "Under all circumstances, therefore, we believe it to be far better to put up with the deformity arising from the superfluous hair, than to endanger the occurrence of a greater evil by attempting its eradication."[52]

CONCERN ABOUT THE "evils" of corrosive or toxic depilatories persisted through the nineteenth century, as markets in commercial hair removers remained unregulated. By the second half of the nineteenth century, some medical practitioners explicitly pondered the need for oversight of commercial cosmetics as a matter of public health. In 1870, the *Medical and Surgical Reporter* held up chemical depilatories as particularly deserving of scrutiny in this regard:

> When it is remembered that precisely those drugs and chemical agents, which are most actively poisonous, enjoy the highest reputation for their beauty-bestowing power, and yet that the manufacture and sale of these agents in secret preparations, engage

millions of dollars of capital annually, in every civilized country, the importance of this inquiry as a
branch of state-medicine, becomes very evident.[53]

Actual legislative oversight of such products, however, was slow
in coming. The U.S. Postal Service and the Federal Trade Commission, which prohibited overt fraud by mail, regulated so-
called cosmetic preparations only to a limited extent. Despite a
growing number of reported injuries and fatalities from commercial depilatories in medical journals, American lawmakers passed
no federal regulations governing the manufacture or sale of hair
removers until the 1912 Sherley Amendment to the 1906 Pure
Food and Drug Act, which prohibited "false and fraudulent therapeutic claims on the labels of patent medicines."[54] Even then, the
amendment prohibited only certain kinds of labeling; it did nothing to test or guarantee the enclosed products.

In the absence of strong legislation regulating the safety and
efficacy of manufactured toiletries, uncertainty bloomed. Purchasers of commercial depilatories had little option but to seek
counsel from external advisors about which products to trust and
which to avoid. As urbanizing Americans relocated away from
the kin and community networks that once helped them to understand and adopt norms of body care, popular newspapers and
magazines began assuming an increasingly advisory role. Advertisers, in particular, took on the task of instructing readers when
and how to use the stream of products emerging from new arts
of manufacture, blanketing growing cities with suggestive copy.[55]
Depilatory manufacturers were exemplary in this respect, insisting on the "equal certainty and safety" of their hair removers,
and warning against the use of "counterfeit" preparations that
might co-opt their hard-earned reputations.[56]

The trajectory of Dr. T. Felix Gouraud provides an illuminating example of the importance of advertising in an emerging industrial order. According to one industry publication, Gouraud
first ventured into the toiletry business in New York in 1839.

Gaining his initial fame through successful sales of a new complexion cream, he soon expanded into depilatory powders. Dr. Felix Gouraud's Poudres Subtile for Uprooting Hair was said to remove hair from "low foreheads, upper lips, arms and hands instantaneously on a single application and positively without injury to the skin." The price for Poudres Subtile was one dollar per bottle—roughly twenty-six dollars in twenty-first-century terms. In the wake of Poudres Subtile, Gouraud's business sailed upward in the United States and Europe through the 1880s.[57]

Gouraud's success in the antebellum depilatory market was tied to his successful manipulation of what would now be referred to as "branding." (The concept of a consumer "brand" did not emerge until the late nineteenth century, when factories began burning their insignia onto shipping barrels like cattle brands.) Gouraud appears to have excelled at establishing a differentiated presence in the burgeoning market in chemical hair removers, manufacturing an image of safety and efficacy alongside the substance of his powder. Advertisements touting the fabricated Dr. Gouraud name—the manufacturer's given name was said to be Felix Trust—appeared in city newspapers through midcentury. He also pioneered the use of celebrity testimonials, including endorsements from famous actresses and opera singers. Gouraud's ability to marshal trust was of particular importance given that the product in question, a caustic depilatory, might cause permanent injury to the user if carelessly made. By 1872, physicians reported that his depilatory was one of the "most common" of all on the market. So successful was the Gouraud label that a long-running legal dispute among Gouraud's relatives over the right to the "Gouraud" name went all the way to the New York Supreme Court.[58]

CRUCIALLY, FELIX TRUST presented Gouraud's Poudres Subtile as bearing not only the ineffable refinement of French culture but also the dreamy allure of the East. Promoting his product as derived from a formula used by the "Queen of Sheba herself,"

Gouraud embodied a trend among early depilatory manufacturers: associating their powders and pastes with the European—and now, Euro-American—imagination of "the Orient."[59] Sheba, whose legendary encounter with King Solomon appears in both the Hebrew Bible and the Qur'an, was a central figure in such Orientalist imagery. Given fresh popularity in the 1840s by Gerard de Nerval's account of his travels in the Levant, *Voyage en Orient* (1843–51), Sheba was a particularly fitting allusion for Gouraud's product: in some versions of the ancient legend, Solomon summoned demons to make a depilatory, called *núra*, which he applied to Sheba's hairy legs.[60]

Such references to the special, perhaps supernatural potency of "Eastern" depilatory compounds, standard fare in elite and popular writings of the nineteenth century, were part of a longer tradition of "Orientalist fantasy," one that, Sarah Berry among others has noted, was "integral to the marketing of cosmetics and self-adornment from the eighteenth-century onward."[61] In colonial America and the early republic, fascination with Eastern mores and customs swelled as British and French soldiers, merchants, and diplomats increased their interventions in the Middle and Far East, and grew along with Americans' own missionary and military ventures in the region. After U.S. Marines marched five hundred miles across what is now the Libyan desert to join the USS *Nautilus*, USS *Hornet*, and USS *Argus* in the bombardment of the port city of Derne in 1805, the role of the Orient in the popular imagination swelled, captured in the famous refrain of the Marine hymn: "to the shores of Tripoli."[62]

Interest in Eastern hair removal practices was a recurrent element of that Orientalist preoccupation, particularly for male travelers.[63] James Atkinson's 1832 English translation of Nah'nah Kulsūm's *Customs and Manners of the Women of Persia* reflects this preoccupation.[64] Atkinson devotes a special explanatory footnote to Kulsūm's brief reference to *núra*. "In eastern countries," Atkinson notes, "the hair under the arms, &c is always removed. Núra is quick lime, or a composition made of it with arsenic, for taking out hairs by the roots." Atkinson's translation also included Kulsūm's report that it was improper for a young girl to use the depilatory, or for a woman to apply it with her own hands, so that "[w]hen women wish to use the núra, they must request a female friend to rub it on."[65] Other writers similarly highlighted the languorous depilation practiced in the Oriental bath. Richard Burton's annotated translation of *Arabian Nights* similarly lingered over the use of depilatories, as did Edward Lane's *Account of the Manners and Customs of the Modern Egyptians* and Alexander Russell's *Natural History of Aleppo.*[66] An essay in the London literary journal *The Casket* featured an account of a "depilatory pomatum" languidly applied to the body; the visitor to the bath was then carefully washed and scrubbed, wrapped in hot linen, and conducted through winding hallways back out of the inner chambers.[67] Andrew Ure described a similar *"oriental rusma"* in his industrial dictionary, stressing that the pomade "yields to nothing in depilatory power"[68] (figure 2.3).

It is difficult to ascertain how influential these depictions may have been in shifting habits in the United States. Certainly no evidence indicates that recurrent references to "Oriental" depilatories led women to remove hair from previously undepilated areas of the body. Yet many if not most commercial depilatory powders and creams, like Gouraud's, alluded to the "Eastern" or "Oriental" origins of their products. These marketing descriptions, along with travelers' and journalists' sensual descriptions of *núra* and *rusma*, proliferated just as the production of depilatories was being relocated from home to factory. In fact, such imaginations of the Orient—seductive, mysterious, and potentially dangerous—gained force as economic activity (like meat production) came increasingly under the practical strictures of factory time. To readers confronting the repetitive piecework and tedious clock time required by industrial manufacturing, images of indulgent Turkish baths filled with unguents probably shimmered with temptation. In their allusions to the mysteries of the Orient, advertisers hinted at access to "spiritual or vital qualities as yet uncontaminated by 'modern' Western thoughts, processes,

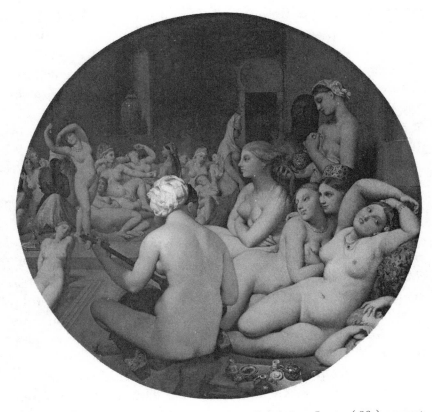

Figure 2.3. *The Turkish Bath* by Jean-Auguste-Dominique Ingres (1862), suggesting Western fascination with "Oriental" depilatory practices. (Courtesy Musée du Louvre.)

and values."[69] So, too, the timeless quality of depictions of Eastern baths may have allowed consumers anxious about packaged compounds to believe that they were made from ancient, well-tested wisdom rather than novel, potentially harmful industrial chemicals. The popularity of references to "Oriental" hair removers in the antebellum period, just as the production of such bodily goods was being relocated from home to factory, suggests this kind of symbolic mediation. Discussions of *núra* and *rusma* helped affix an exotic, preindustrial aura to new manufactured goods.[70]

Indeed, some critics worried that advertisers' mystified images of the Orient were acting to obscure awareness of the potentially injurious effects of depilatory chemicals. The *Workingman's Advocate* complained as much in 1830: "[U]nsuspecting delicate females" find themselves "lulled into the belief that these [arsenic and pearl-white depilatories] are harmless, because they are graced by pretty names, Oriental, Itilian [sic], or French." But in truth, such "chemicals of the toilette . . . very materially assist the messenger of death. There is scarce a cosmetic that is not a deleterious and destructive poison."[71] Another strong critique of commercial preparations concluded that women would be better off consulting recipe manuals and making their own toiletries, which would "certainly be more safe, and we believe far more beneficial than the patent nostrums."[72] Likewise, the 1834 *Toilette of Health, Beauty, and Fashion* recommended homemade compounds of parsley water, acacia juice, and gum of ivy, or milk thistle mixed with oil.[73] Andrew Ure recommended tempering the "causticity" of store-bought hair-removing pomades by adding a bit of "starch or rye flour" from the kitchen.[74]

Such advice points to an ambivalent process of accommodation, as Americans shifted from using familiar, handcrafted preparations to purchasing commodities produced at a distance. Ambivalence is understandable, as the market revolution at once expanded the array of available off-the-shelf goods and rendered purchasers newly vulnerable to obscure and unregulated processes of production. While the shift from homemade depilatories to those concocted at remote perfumeries was surely one of the more modest features of the nation's turbulent transition from agrarianism to industrial manufacturing, it did require an uncommonly visceral absorption of that larger sea change: applying the products of industry directly to one's face. In this sense, the seeming banality of hair removal helped veiled the significance of the transformation: women's active incorporation of an emerging economic system. Like other elements of daily life, care of the body was entwined in a strange new industrial order.[75]

BEARDED WOMEN
AND DOG-FACED MEN

Darwin's Great Denudation

EVEN AS INDUSTRIAL and geopolitical change brought heightened attention to packaged depilatory powders, disdain for visible body hair remained relatively contained through the first half of the nineteenth century, an attitude considered specific to American "Indians." Other than the men of science busily establishing racial differences in hair growth, the perfumers and druggists pushing treatments for low foreheads or side whiskers, and sideshow barkers seeking to profit from the exhibition of spectacularly hairy individuals, few Americans at midcentury appear to have given much thought to body hair.

After 1871, however, attitudes began to shift. With the publication of Charles Darwin's *Descent of Man*, perspectives on the relations between "man" and "brute" received a startling jolt.[1] Darwinian frameworks and vocabularies, spread by scientific and medical experts and by the popular press, came to exercise enormous influence on American ideas about hair, fur, wool, and the differences—such as they were—between them. After *Descent*, dwindling numbers of Americans would attribute visible differences in body hair to divine design or to the relative balance of bile, blood, and phlegm. Instead, differences in hair type and amount came to be described as effects of evolutionary forces: the tangible result of competitive selection. Moreover, the same traditions of comparative anatomy that helped to launch evolutionary theory provoked ongoing interest in the scientific analysis of body hair. Although these diverse experts never spoke with one voice on the significance of body hair, collectively they succeeded in pathologizing "excessive" hair growth. By the dawn of the twentieth century, hairiness had been established as a sign of sexual, mental, and criminal deviance.

ALTHOUGH DARWIN HINTED in his 1859 introduction to the *Origin of Species* that the book would shed light on the contentious subject of "man and his origins," not until 1871's *Descent of Man* did he seek to explain both how man was "descended from some pre-existing form" and how apparent variations in physical characteristics came to be: why some bodies are darker or furrier or smaller than others, and so on.[2]

Body hair played a pivotal (and underappreciated) role in both explanations. The evolutionary ideas often said to have been "discovered" by Darwin were actually pieced together from many sources; chief among those sources were earlier comparative studies of hair.[3] Among the many details from his encyclopedic notes that Darwin included in *Descent* are accounts of the eradication of eyebrows in South America and Africa; of the monetary value (twenty shillings) accorded to the loss of a beard in Anglo-Saxon law; and of the Fuegian Islanders' threat to a particular young missionary ("far from a hairy man") that they would "strip him naked, and pluck the hairs from his face and body."[4] Darwin took many of these examples from two American sources: Catlin's two-volume 1841 ethnography of the manners and customs of North American Indians and Gould's massive 1869 survey of Civil War soldiers.[5]

If Darwin wished merely to describe the influence of the aesthetic in human evolution—the role of "beauty" once noted by James Cowles Prichard—he might have focused on any number of characteristics: eye size, hip-to-shoulder ratio, limb length. (Twenty-first-century evolutionary biologists analyze all these features and more.) Hairiness, however, forced particularly

challenging questions about man's relations to his primate fore-
bears, as Darwin, like earlier naturalists, well realized. On the
one hand, the very presence of hair would seem to fortify the
claim that man is "descended from some ape-like creature."[6] As
Darwin reasoned, "From the presence of the woolly hair . . . we
may infer that man is descended from some animal which was
born hairy and remained so during life."[7] And yet, that same
thin scattering of hairs posed a rather inconvenient truth for the
theory of natural selection, since the detriments of man's relative *hairlessness* was readily apparent to anyone who had suffered through a clammy English winter. As Darwin explained,
"The loss of hair is an inconvenience and probably an injury to
man even under a hot climate, for he is thus exposed to sudden
chills, especially during wet weather."[8] Darwin concluded that
man's "more or less complete absence of hair" reveals the limits of the arguments he laid out in the *Origin of Species.*[9] "No
one supposes that the nakedness of the skin is any direct advantage to man, so that his body cannot have been divested of hair
through natural selection."[10]

The problem Darwin faced in the *Descent*, then, was to make
sense of characteristics that were useless at best and injurious or
downright lethal at worst, given natural selection's overarching
insistence that advantageous variations persist over others. This
dilemma was embodied most fully in what Darwin called the
great "denudation of mankind"—man's loss of hairy covering.[11]
Resolving this dilemma compelled Darwin to unfurl his controversial companion to the theory of natural selection: sexual selection. Thus the explicit goal of the latter sections of *Descent*, the
chapters that discuss the inheritance of disadvantageous characteristics, is to show that such selection, "continued through many
generations," can produce effects on bodily form and appearance.[12] Ultimately, Darwin attributed most of the differences of
concern to his nineteenth-century readers—why some creatures
were stronger or larger or more colorful than others—to the action of sexual selection. As he concluded in the *Descent*, "of all the

causes which have led to the differences in external appearance between the races of man, and to a certain extent between man and the lower animals, sexual selection has been by far the most efficient."[13]

DARWIN'S ADVOCACY OF sexual selection—and specifically its role in explaining man's relative hairlessness—drove a wedge between Darwin and his longtime collaborator, Alfred Russel Wallace.[14] Like Darwin's *Descent of Man*, Wallace's major book on human evolution, his 1870 *Contributions to the Theory of Natural Selection*, wrestled with how to accommodate seemingly useless or disadvantageous characteristics within the confines of the theory of natural selection. Chief among these troublesome characteristics was what Wallace called the absence of "hairy covering" in man. Other characteristics were similarly inexplicable, Wallace proposed, but perhaps not to "an equal degree."[15] Considering man's hairless condition against the backdrop of other similarly perplexing phenomena led Wallace to conclude that man's nakedness demonstrated "the agency of some other power than the law of the survival of the fittest." In his view, hairlessness could be explained in no other way. As Wallace put it, a "superior intelligence has guided the development of man in a definite direction, and for a special purpose," by means of "more subtle agencies than we are acquainted with."[16]

More steadfast evolutionists quickly jumped on this point. In one 1870 lecture, the Devonshire naturalist and theologian T. R. R. Stebbing lambasted Wallace for failing to recognize the capacious meanings of "utility" in the struggle for existence. "[W]hat is selected through being useful in one direction may incidentally become useful in another," Stebbing argued. "Had [Wallace] employed his usual ingenuity on the question of man's hairless skin, he might have seen the possibility of its 'selection' through its superior beauty or the health attached to superior cleanliness."[17] Stebbing further mocked Wallace's claims by ridiculing the idea of God as some sort of primordial cosmetologist:

[I]t is surprising that he should picture to himself a superior intelligence plucking the hair from the backs
of savage men . . . in order that the descendents of the
poor shorn wretches might, after many deaths from
cold and damp, in the course of many generations take
to tailoring and to dabbling in bricks and mortar.[18]

Such trappings of civility, Stebbing insisted, are "nothing more
nor less than part and parcel of natural selection."[19]

Recognizing body hair as the key point of contention, Darwin
zeroed in on both Wallace's statements and Stebbing's critique.
In *Descent*, Darwin echoed Stebbing's dismissal of Wallace, and
reasserted the absurdity of thinking that hairlessness was God's
way to force early men "to raise themselves in the scale of civilization through the practice of various arts."[20] Hairlessness had an
explanation, to be sure—but its explanation was earthly rather
than divine: men's election of "superior beauty and cleanliness."
In the midst of his most important statement on human evolution, Darwin narrated his break with Wallace as a disagreement
over the origins and purposes of body hair: where Wallace saw divine determination, Darwin saw individual choice.

"CHOICE" FOR DARWIN did not necessarily involve anything one
might now consider deliberation or calculation on the part of the
chooser. "As far as sexual selection is concerned," Darwin wrote,
"all that is required is that choice should be exerted."[21] Even if the
individual member of a species does not intend to produce consequences on the bodies of his remote descendants, consequences
there will be. As Darwin put it, "[A]n effect would be produced,
independently of any wish or expectation on the part of the men
who preferred certain women to others."[22] He repeated this point
for emphasis: "[U]nconscious selection would come into action."[23] The potential for *unconscious* selection is key, since, again,
the theory was developed to account for those features, such as
hairlessness, which were, in Darwin's words, "of no service" to

animals "in their ordinary habits of life."[24] Man's "partial loss of hair," Darwin argued, is thus one of those "innumerable strange characters . . . modified through sexual selection." It is not hard to believe, he assured, that a characteristic as injurious as hairlessness had been acquired in this way; for "we know that this is the case with the plumes of some birds, and with the horns of some stags." Although unwieldy horns and plumes might obstruct key activities such as eating or escaping predators, females might find them attractive enough that, over time, an aberrant trait might eventually become widespread.[25]

But herein lies the problem. Quite unlike the fancy horns of the Irish elk or the resplendent plumage of the Bower-bird, human hairlessness is, according to Darwin's own examples, a *cultivated* characteristic, the product of meticulous care. "[M]en of the beardless races," Darwin himself wrote, "take infinite pains in eradicating every hair from their faces, as something odious, whilst the men of the bearded races feel the greatest pride in their beards," and care for them accordingly.[26] While sexual selection might well explain characteristics that seem to confer no other evolutionary advantage, the question remains as to exactly how one confers the effects of ornamental grooming on one's offspring.

So how did early humans lose their hairy covering, if not through the inheritance of acquired characteristics—the very principle, proposed by French naturalist Jean-Baptiste Lamarck, that Darwin is generally credited with refuting? At this key juncture of the *Descent of Man*, Darwin skirted the Lamarckian implications of his explanation by employing the passive voice:

> As far as the extreme intricacy of the subject permits us to judge, it appears that our male ape-like progenitors acquired their beards as an ornament to charm or excite the opposite sex, and transmitted them to man as he now exists. The females apparently were first denuded of hair in like manner as a sexual ornament.[27]

How that "first denudation" happened, occurring as it did when denudation was of no particular service, remains murky.

THE MURKINESS OF this narrative did not elude critics. One particularly witty 1871 satire by Richard Grant White—Shakespeare scholar, journalist, and father of the architect Stanford White—highlighted the problems posed by Darwin's account of the great denudation by retelling the story of man's descent from the point of view of gorillas (figure 3.1).[28]

The story of *The Fall of Man*, the gorilla narrator tells us, began "[l]ong ago," when, through a "deplorable freak of nature," one male gorilla was born deformed, almost entirely without hair. But the gorilla was not shunned; rather, many of the young female gorillas, showing the "unaccountable caprice of their sex," developed "a hankering after this young fellow." He declared himself "not a marrying gorilla" and announced to his crowd of yearning females that "until he found one whose coat was even softer and slighter than his own, he [w]ould remain a bachelor."[29] A particularly lovesick female gorilla grew determined to win his favor. Day and night, she fretted over how to rid herself of her "disgusting coat of coarse hair."[30]

One fateful day the lonely, lovesick gorilla sat down against a tree to muse on her problems, without realizing that the tree was coated with thick, half-dried gum. While she sat there pining, "[t]he hair on the outside of her arm [became] imbedded in the gum, which, drying as she leaned, held her fast."[31] As there were no other gorillas nearby to help free her, the young female decided that she had no option other than to rip herself free: "Summoning all her fortitude and her force, she threw herself forward and fell upon the ground with a scream that might have been heard afar off, for she had torn out by the roots every hair that had touched the tree."[32] Once her pain passed, the gorilla worried that she might now be even more repulsive to the object of her affection, given the raw, bare patch on her arm. But before long, the gorilla narrator continues,

THE FALL OF MAN:

OR,

THE LOVES OF THE GORILLAS.

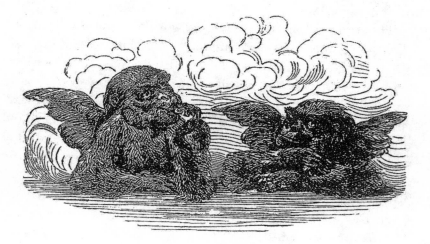

A POPULAR SCIENTIFIC LECTURE UPON THE

Darwinian Theory of Development by Sexual Selection.

BY A LEARNED GORILLA.

Edited by the Author of

"THE NEW GOSPEL OF PEACE."

Figure 3.1. Richard Grant White satirizes Darwin's explanation of the relative hairlessness of "man" (1871).

[S]he was led from despair to hope by a strange way of thinking which man calls reason. . . . [S]he thought that if the object of her love longed for a female with a coat softer and finer and sparser than his own, he might, . . . therefore (but who of us can tell what *therefore* means?), possibly like one better yet who had no hairy coat at all.[33]

THUS SHE BEGAN. She remained hidden in seclusion as she returned to the gum tree week after week, until she had denuded her entire body with this "new depilatory." When her "sacrificial transformation" was finally complete and she revealed herself to the male gorilla, he was totally enamored by the smooth limbs that "all unknown to him, had suffered such torment for his delight."[34] She continued her self-treatments with the gum tree, and also continued to conceal the "artifice [to which] she owed her hairless skin."[35] When she later gave birth to a relatively hairless boy, the narrative concludes, the baby "inherited from his mother those strange thoughts, 'therefore' and 'I am ashamed.'"[36]

The *Fall of Man* made comically explicit what Darwin, Wallace, and Stebbing left implicit: stories about body hair reveal larger assumptions about suffering, choice, and what ultimately separates "man" from other animals. Whether a "superior intelligence" plucked the hair from savage men to drive them to tailoring and brick-laying, or whether some early ape determined the course of this "sacrificial transformation," explications of humans' relative hairlessness conveyed implicit social values.

AMERICAN THEOLOGIANS, WELL aware of the profound implications of Darwin's ideas, largely ignored or outright rejected the claims made in *Descent* through much of the century. But already by the mid-1870s, American botanists, geologists, and ethnologists were adopting evolutionary frameworks and applying them to their work. Coinciding with sociologists' interest in the

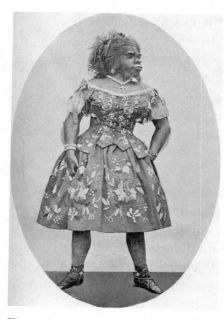

Figure 3.2. An undated depiction of the mid-nineteenth-century performer Julia Pastrana, reproduced in *The Living Races of Mankind* (1900).

historical implications of competitive forces, Darwinian ideas were absorbed into American thought more broadly.[57]

The influence of evolutionary vocabularies is manifest in post-*Descent* representations of extraordinarily hairy people, many of whom were displayed in nineteenth-century circuses and freak shows as "dog-faced men" or "bearded ladies."[58] The celebrated midcentury performer Julia Pastrana provides a case in point (figure 3.2). Prior to the Civil War, exhibition handbills characterized the famously hairy Pastrana as a "hybrid" of woman and "Ourang-Outang," a member of a "race of savages" from Mexico, or the offspring of an Indian and a bear. Said to possess exquisite moral and temperamental faculties, Pastrana allegedly represented that point "where man's bestial attributes terminate and . . . those that are *Divine* begin."[59] Yet after Darwin expressed interest in Pastrana in his 1868 *Variation of Animals and Plants under Domestication* (describing her as a "remarkably fine woman" with a "gorilla-like appearance"), she and other similarly hairy individuals were renarrated as "splendid illustration[s] of Mr. Darwin's theory."[40] A photograph of a thirteen-year-old girl in Vienna with "skin more like a fur than anything else," one weekly concluded, might be used to illustrate new editions of Darwin's work.[41] The girl noted earlier, Krao, similarly was exhibited as a "living specimen" of the ancestral ties between men and monkeys.[42] Discussing the case of a "dog-faced boy," one physician noted that he had cause to doubt whether such patients were "member[s] of the human family."[43]

Evolutionary understandings of body hair were not limited to the exceptionally hairy people discussed and displayed as "freaks." Along with a plethora of popular cartoons conveying Darwin's ideas (or Darwin himself [figure 3.3]) through images of hairy monkeys, more mundane representations of hair also began to reflect evolutionary frameworks.[44] Our "hairs," reported one popular weekly in 1873, "are appendages of the skin, contributing to its defence," their thickness "regulated by the law of Nature." Hair is no "less useful because it is ornamental."[45] Hair's status as an artifact of selective pressures was also affirmed by allusions to the similarities between man and beast; in the last quarter of the nineteenth century, the once-controversial claim that "hoofs and hair are homologous appendages" became largely taken for granted.[46] The term "well-groomed," for instance, first coined in 1886, referred evenly well to horse or man.

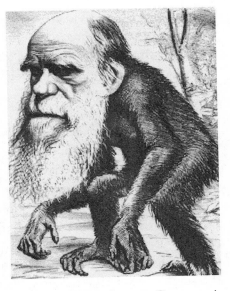

Figure 3.3. A popular post-*Descent* caricature of Darwin as a "Venerable Orangoutang," first published in the satirical magazine the *Hornet* (1871).

AS EVOLUTIONARY IDEAS about hair seeped into everyday conversation, scientific and medical experts grew more concerned with what became known as "excessive" hair growth. Aesthetic concerns were transmuted into questions of evolutionary fitness. In 1878, seven years after the publication of *Descent* and one year after the first meeting of the newly formed American Dermatological Association, a Danish physician proposed a new disease category for the individual, "homo hirsutus," said to suffer from excessive hair: *hypertrichosis*.[47] Subsequent practitioners began to diagnose disease when hair was found to be abnormal in location, quantity, or quality. As one physician working on the subject succinctly stated, "hypertrichosis is defined as an unnatural growth of hair."[48]

But which hair, exactly, was to be considered unnatural? Predictably, the new diagnostic category produced a recurrent dilemma for clinical practice: distinguishing pathological levels of hairiness from ordinary hair growth. As with nymphomania (excessive sexual desire), alcoholism (excessive drunkenness), and other diseases first labeled in the nineteenth century, the criteria used to diagnose hypertrichosis were flexible and contested.[49] Experts disagreed, for instance, on how to demarcate the soft downy hairs known as *lanugo* (widely considered "normal") from the "strong," dark growths thought to be indicative of disease; in the words of one physician, "the one verges into the other almost imperceptibly."[50] Making matters more difficult, experts trying to pin down a single definition of excessive hair identified racial variations in both hair growth and perceptions of that growth. Some reported a tendency for hypertrichosis in patients "of Jewish and Celtic extraction," others in patients of Russian or Italian descent.[51] Still others justified the exclusion of "negroes" from their studies of hair growth by insisting that a "deficiency of secondary hair is frequent in these people as compared to Caucasians."[52] Meanwhile, the fine amounts of facial hair on the "Mongolian, the American Indian and the Malay," one specialist pointed out, might lead these peoples to find grotesque the prodigious quantity of hair "that is ordinarily found on the faces of Europeans."[53]

Despite such diagnostic confusion, sorting normal from excessive hair became a pressing concern for late-nineteenth-century experts, who approached visible hair, particularly visible facial hair on women, as a crucial if often confusing marker of ill health. Post-Darwinian medical texts were rife with detailed classifying schema, designed to assist physicians in diagnosis. One dermatologist carefully delineated six types of hairy patients who might appear requesting treatment, from the woman with "a very fine white lanugo on the upper lip and sides of the cheeks" (which "is noticeable only to herself and should not be treated"), through the brunette with a short fine mustache (which "adds a certain artistic picture which is natural for that type of individual" and should also be left untreated), up to the patient who "shows coarse, stiff, long hairs" that "occupy the same regions as the male beard" ("This condition is a real indication for treatment").[54] In especially complicated cases, the dermatologist explained, the presentation of the woman patient's "male secondary sex characteristics" is "shown by her expression as well as the distribution and coarseness of the hair."[55] When nature was functioning properly, experts after *Descent* presumed, men had body hair, and women did not.

More precisely, young women did not have body hair. Consistent with evolutionary arguments concerning sexual selection, physicians typically proclaimed hairiness to be of medical significance only for premenopausal women. Reproductive pair bonding was the goal. As physician Adolph Brand explained, the practitioner's primary encounter with hypertrichosis was among women between the ages of eighteen and thirty-five, "[t]his being the period of a woman's life during which her physical charms receive her greatest attention."[56] Another expert suggested that the "great majority" of cases of hypertrichosis affected women between the ages of twenty and thirty.[57] The age of the patient affected not only medical diagnosis but also medical treatment. One physician reported a colleague's therapeutic principles: "While his indications are humane and even chivalrous to female sufferers under twenty-five years, his advice [is] not to yield to the entreaties of a married woman." For patients over forty-five, the physician advised forgoing all treatment.[58]

Body hair's role in sexual and reproductive fitness was further emphasized by medical reports of patients' subjective experiences of hairiness. One of the few women physicians recorded in the related literature, Dr. Henrietta Johnson, described "one beautiful and attractive woman" who "would not marry, lest the hairy tendency which had made her own life a wretched one, and which she had tried by every known artifice to conceal, might be transmitted to her female offspring."[59] (Johnson did not elaborate further on the "hairy tendency.") Emphasizing young women's deep, instinctual desire for hairlessness, dermatologist Ernest McEwen similarly insisted that women themselves yearned for effective treatment.

> The woman afflicted feels herself an object of repulsion to the opposite sex, and as a result, set apart from the normal members of her own sex. She realizes that she bears a stigma of the male and that she does not run true to the female type; therefore, every female instinct in her demands that the thing which marks her as different from other women be removed.[60]

Although they could not agree on clear standards of "normal" hairiness, physicians remained assured that for young women, abnormal hair growth ran counter to "female instinct."

ONGOING ATTEMPTS TO quantify and classify hair growth reflected broader efforts to discern exactly what "excessive" hair might signal about its possessor. Born of the same anthropometric traditions of comparative measurement and observation that gave rise to Darwin's theories of variation, diverse groups of investigators began counting hairs as a way to engage wider social and political concerns. Their analyses were part of a significant cultural shift ongoing in the late nineteenth century: one moving "deviance" from its traditional location in criminal law to the domain of medical science.[61]

Particularly influential in this regard was the young field of study known as "sexology," which approached most so-called sexual abnormalities not as perversions of a person's object of desire (as later concepts of homosexuality would imply) but as reversals or confusions of one's own sex role. Sexual deviance was defined largely by the observation of "virile" traits or habits among women or "effeminate" traits or habits among men. Early sexologists in Europe and North America thus focused on the observation of such traits and habits in individuals, enumerating and categorizing their case reports into various types of sexual "inversion."[62] The most influential sexologists of the late nineteenth century—Havelock Ellis, Magnus Hirschfeld, Richard von Krafft-Ebing, and Albert Moll—concentrated these observations on "secondary sexual characteristics." Secondary sexual characteristics, Krafft-Ebing explained, were those "bodily and psychical" traits, such as facial hair or breasts, that develop "only during the period of puberty" and help "differentiate the two sexes."[63]

Of course, the very concept of secondary sexual characteristics implied the possibility of slippage between "primary" and "secondary" identifications, and sexologists readily acknowledged the myriad difficulties of aligning the two. Sexologists further determined that inversions, forms of sexual deviance, were often subtle, complex, and even contradictory. "Observation teaches that the pure type of the man or the woman is often enough missed by nature," Krafft-Ebing wrote, "that is to say that certain secondary male characteristics are found in woman and vice versa." Examples might include "men with an inclination for female occupations (embroidery, toilet, etc.)" and "women with a decided predilection for manly sports."[64] The complexities of sexual classifications were amplified, sexologists believed, by racial variation in secondary sexual characteristics: "The higher the anthropological development of the race, the stronger these contrasts between man and woman, and vice versa."[65] As sexologists sought to distinguish the truly "pathological" inversion from a mild fondness for embroidery or boxing, sorting genuinely "feminine" characteristics from the "masculine" became paramount.

Body hair, considered one of the leading secondary sex characteristics, presented particular challenges to this effort. To begin, hair growth was troublingly unpredictable, varying from individual to individual, from life stage to life stage, and from season to season. Moreover, hair's connection to sexual inversion remained uncertain, even as sexologists meticulously examined patients' bodies for signs of "unusual" hair growth.[66] The clinician and activist Magnus Hirschfeld, assessing the body hair of more than 500 men, claimed a link between sexual roles and relative amounts of hair. He determined that the beards of 132 of the "inverted" men in his study were "'sparser than in average men'"; another 98 "had no body hair at all, 78 had unusually fine body hair, and 176 had body hair less dense than in average males."[67] Those findings were disputed by Krafft-Ebing, whose scrutiny of the face, trunk, pubic region, and extremities found no similar correspondence between hairiness and inversion.[68] For Krafft-Ebing, it was less hair itself than attitudes toward hair that indicated sexual abnormality. To illustrate the point, Krafft-Ebing described the case of a "silent, retiring, unsocial, and sullen" man who arrived at an asylum at the age of twenty-three. Over his years in the institution, "his personality became completely feminine."[69] Along with a request for women's clothing and a transfer to the female wing of the hospital (where he might find protection from "men that wished to violate him"), the patient demanded the application of an "'Oriental Hair-Remover'" in order that "no one may doubt" his true sex. For Krafft-Ebing, the patient's manifest distaste for his own body hair, rather than his relative degree of pilosity, was the real indication of "deviance."[70]

As equivocal as they were on the relationship between body hair and male sexual inversion, early sexologists were equally mystified by hair's relationship to female inversion. Some insisted that hair growth in a "masculine" pattern suggested a deeper confusion of sexual role; others reported that women with flowing beards tended to exhibit exemplary "feminine" characteristics in all other respects. The most influential and authoritative sexologist in America in the 1890s, British physician Havelock Ellis, reflected this wider ambivalence about the meanings of hair. Ellis, an honorary member of the Chicago Academy of Medicine, member of the Medico-Legal Society of New York, and vice president of the International Medical and Legal Congress of New York, confronted the relations between hairiness and female sexuality directly in his first American publication. In 1895, he declared it "a mistake to suppose that bearded women approach the masculine type," particularly because female inverts may appear without "any trace of a beard or moustache."[71] Two years later, however, Ellis revisited that confident assertion, allowing that one of the female inverts he had studied did indeed have an "unusual growth of hair on the legs." Writing in the first English-language medical textbook on the subject of sexual inversion, he further proposed that "[a] woman physician in the United States, who knows many inverts of her own sex, tells me that she has observed this growth of hair on the legs."[72] Whether visibly hairy legs or upper lips indicated female deviance remained open to debate.

ALTHOUGH SEXOLOGISTS COULD not reach consensus on the links between body hair and sexual inversion, they readily joined late-nineteenth-century criminologists, alienists, and dermatologists in asserting an association between heavy hair growth and mental illness. This association was not novel; hairiness had long been considered a sign of lunacy. Medieval iconography, for instance, routinely used shaggy skin to exemplify the disturbance of penitents experiencing holy madness. Beginning in the twelfth century, the biblical Nebuchadnezzar—the Babylonian king whose humiliating descent into madness left him living like an animal in the wilderness—was depicted as covered in hair. (figure 3.4)[73]

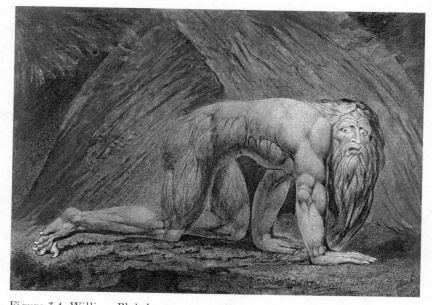

Figure 3.4. William Blake's 1795 portrayal of the mad king Nebuchadnezzar as covered with thick hair. (Courtesy of Tate Britain.)

Yet as lunacy, like sexuality, became the object of scientific rather than theological or criminal investigation, examining differences in hair became a favored method of medical classification.[74] Already in the 1840s, the lawyer and slavery advocate Peter Browne was collecting specimens of hair from mental hospitals in order to identify the shape and form characteristic of insanity. In the sensational 1851 lunacy trial of Warder Cresson, a Philadelphia Quaker whose circumcision and conversion to Judaism prompted his family to declare him mentally incompetent, Browne served as a witness, displaying to the jury "many hundred specimens of hair from five lunatic hospitals." Based on a microscopic analysis of a hair root sample from Cresson (which Browne said showed a white, transparent, regularly shaped structure at the end, unlike the dark, distorted, and irregularly shaped structure allegedly "characteristic of insanity"), Browne concluded in favor of Cresson's sanity.[75] Browne's findings were widely circulated, and once the influential German physician Rudolf Virchow posited a relationship between hair growth and neurosis based on his own observations, other investigators confidently asserted the connections between emotional, mental, and "nervous" disturbances and unusual hair growth.[76] One 1872 treatise linked pathologies in female hair growth to social pathologies in a number of instances, as in the case of one young woman patient—with pronounced moustache and beard—whose "mother was insane," her sister "in a lunatic asylum," and another sister "nearly raving with neuralgia."[77] An 1893 study of 272 cases of insanity in white women noted that not only did insane women present excessive facial hair more frequently than the sane, but their hairs were also "thicker and stiffer," more "closely resembl[ing] those of the inferior races."[78] In his own book-length study of criminality, Ellis cited five different experts when claiming that the single "most characteristic physical feature" of criminal women, particularly "women guilty of infanticide," was their "remarkable abundance of hair." Ellis postulated that abundant hair growth, like criminal violence and "strong sexual instincts," might be correlated with exceptional "animal vigour."[79]

TRANSGRESSIVE WOMEN HAVE been accused of possessing animal spirits for centuries, of course.[80] But the meanings of animality changed after Darwin. And, as diverse communities of women began challenging established sexual roles more intensely—pushing for access to education and the vote, breaking into occupations once exclusively male, lobbying for the right to control their own wages—scientific attention to purportedly innate sexual inequalities proliferated. The lurking threat of degeneracy conveyed in the wake of the *Descent of Man*, paired with heightened expert concern with the meaning of secondary sex characteristics, gave hair renewed cultural weight. By the 1920s, when aversion to body hair reached unprecedented levels of intensity, best-selling authors confidently asserted that superfluous hair indicated "a 'throw back' tendency," whereby "for some inscrutable reason Nature brings forth a condition simulating that which existed in her first attempts to transform a hairy animal into a comparatively hairless man."[81] With body hair, particularly women's facial hair, newly yoked to evolutionary atavism, individual pathology, sexual inversion, and mental illness, efforts to remove hair boomed. Experts and laypeople alike began devoting fresh energy to "remedy[ing] the evil" of superfluous hair.[82]

[4]

"SMOOTH, WHITE, VELVETY SKIN"

X-Ray Salons and Social Mobility

THE FASCINATION WITH body hair fertilized by theories of sexual selection blossomed in the opening decades of the twentieth century. Women's body hair, in particular, attracted fervent attention. Physician after physician described the severe depression, self-imposed seclusion, and nausea common to women "afflicted" with heavy hair growth—particularly hair on the face. In 1913, one recalled a typical patient who "gave up a very lucrative position, shunned all her acquaintances, refused to go out unless heavily veiled, and slowly drifted into true melancholia" due to her hairiness.[1] "Subjects of this growth are notably sensitive and depressed," said another in the *Journal of the American Medical Association*, as well as "embittered, melancholy and resentful." Often, he continued, patients "asserted that death was preferable to the life of embarrassment they had to live."[2] Other physicians similarly described patients who considered (or accomplished) escaping their misery through suicide.[3]

Physicians were not exaggerating the depth of women's distress. American women's mounting apprehension about body hair is evident in their letters to popular magazine editors, beauty experts, and health advisors. One 26-year-old from Pittsburgh began one such letter by noting plaintively that "people have told me, I am pretty." But "of late," she continued, "a heavy growth of hair has appeared all over my face. It so embarrasses me that I have begun to shrink from contact with anyone."[4] Although hair

75

on the face and neck—those areas of the body most difficult to conceal—remained of greatest concern, women also began expressing embarrassment or shame about hair elsewhere on the body. An unmarried woman from Franklin, Pennsylvania, described herself as "handicapped" by hair on her "face and body,"[5] while a physician's wife from Pelion, South Carolina, described her arms and legs as "so hairy they are bad looking."[6] Their words suggest painful struggles to comply with intensified expectations of hairlessness.

Several developments converged to shape these expectations, including not only the rapid growth of print advertising and newly revealing fashions in clothing but also changing gender and sexual roles and intensifying emphasis on racialized ideals of hygiene. As ever, body hair was a ready repository for wider social and political concerns. But equally crucial to emerging norms of hair management was the diffusion of "modern," salon-based therapies, including electrolysis, diathermy, and x-radiation. The scientific aura enveloping those novel techniques of hair removal—an aura touted by professional physicians no less than nonmedical beauty specialists—helped give new practices of hair removal mass appeal.

AT THE TURN of the twentieth century, the status of women, particularly native-born white women, was the subject of tremendous professional and popular concern. The gathering momentum of the suffrage movement, increasingly frank and public conversation about contraception, declining rates of reproduction among college-educated women, and the growing visibility of wage-earning women all contributed to a volatile mixture of confusion, anger, and hope about the "new woman" and her challenge to sexual roles.[7] In the midst of this tumult, women's body hair was a multivalent symbol. For critics of changing sexual roles, visible body hair on women served as tangible evidence of a surfeit of manliness. As women who pushed for voting rights and access to jobs and education were depicted as sexually inverted, so, too, were they depicted as hairy. One New York physician, Herbert Claiborne, proposed in 1914 a single explanation for excessive hairiness, lesbianism, and the "violent and vicious" activities of suffragists and businesswomen: the exaggeration of "masculine traits" in their "structural and psychic being."[8] Visible body hair, like women's smoking, drinking, and paid labor outside the home, became a ready mark of the new woman's "excessive" sexual, political, and economic independence.[9] At the same time, body hair offered women a tool for experimental self-fashioning: a curious young person might try removing some hair as a temporary rebellion, and then let it grow back as needed. Like cosmetic use, women could adopt new practices of hair removal as a transient test of modern styles.[10] Pushed from opposite directions by women seeking new social roles and by critics of those roles, aversion to women's body hair spread rapidly.

That aversion was augmented by the growing influence of the hygiene movement. The movement's focus on hygienic health was overtly racial; whiteness was linked to social "fitness." Concern about the racial "in-betweenness" of new immigrant groups (seen as not *quite* white) was mirrored in concern about impurity and pollution in other domains, such as sexual conduct, housekeeping, and personal care. Industry organizations such as the Cleanliness Institute offered prodigious advice on hygienic behavior, including meticulous schedules for bodily upkeep. Actively seeking to extend scientific ands medical authority over daily habits, a generation of hygiene experts stressed the importance of segregating oneself from organic life and its polluting microbes. This preoccupation with spotlessness was made manifest in period advertisements: voluptuous flesh and visible hair yielded to clean, athletic figures, whose smooth, sanitized whiteness was crucial to their virtue.[11]

Increased investment in hygiene dovetailed with changes in dress. Prompted by women's demands for less restrictive clothing and enabled by the distribution of cheaper, mass-produced fabric, middle-class women's clothing began drawing attention to previously concealed parts of the body. Hemlines began to rise noticeably around 1910; by 1915, they had reached midcalf, and by 1927 they brushed just below the knee. Sleeve length, too, began to retract over the same twenty-year period, slowly "unveiling" the female form.[12] These trends in fashion, numerous commentators noted, seemed to reflect larger trends in thought. Edward Bok, influential editor of the *Ladies Home Journal*, expressed dismay characteristic of the time when declaring that new women "are donning masculinity, not only in their garments, but in their ideas."[13]

As progressive women began asserting new habits of bodily self-determination and styles in women's clothing revealed more and more hair-bearing areas of the body, more and more American women began to remove visible hair from their arms and armpits. Where once hair removal among most non-Native women was confined to upper lips, foreheads, and hands, now arms, armpits, chests, and even legs became targets for treatment. (Thick stockings continued to be widely used to veil hair on calves and ankles exposed by rising hemlines.) Untreated skin that had once been covered by clothing now threatened to divulge subtle evidence of atavism, as Prufrock laments in T. S. Eliot's famous 1917 poem:

> *I have known the arms already, known them all—*
> *Arms that are braceleted and white and bare*
> *(But in the lamplight, downed with light brown hair!)*[14]

The importance of hair-free limbs was underscored throughout the burgeoning number of magazines directed to women readers.[15] *Harper's Bazaar* alone displayed a fivefold increase in the number of advertisements for hair removal products over the period from 1915 to 1919, outstripping any similar increase in other personal care products.[16] Other popular magazines targeted to white women—*Screen Secrets*, *Style Magazine*, *Vogue*, and so on—began similarly promoting hairless armpits, arms, faces, and necks as essential to feminine beauty. A series of advertisements for the depilatory Del-a-tone insisted that its use "is necessary so long as sleeveless gowns and sheer fabrics for sleeves are worn."[17] A promotion for a depilatory manufactured by the De Miracle Chemical Company warned more seriously that America "May Become a Nation of Bearded Women" unless consumers acted quickly.[18] Advice columns and popular beauty books further underscored the necessity of the new practices.[19]

Thus, even as fashion and custom allowed some women unprecedented freedom of movement, new forms of self-regulation and constraint were coming into being.[20] In a remarkably short time, historian Peter Stearns summarizes, "body hair became disgusting" to middle-class American women, its removal a way "to separate oneself from cruder people, lower class and immigrant."[21] As psychologist Knight Dunlap recalled the shift in a 1917 address, at first only a few "women removed their axillary hair, others did not. A little later, the practice of removing the hair became practically universal, and now the hair is seldom seen."[22] By 1938, one expert declared without sarcasm that any publicly visible hair not on a woman's scalp was rightly considered "excessive."[23]

IN THE 1920S AND 1930S, the woman seeking to rid herself of hair had an array of temporary, flawed solutions at her disposal. Abrasives such as fine-grained pumice stone, sugar-paste solutions, or so-called Velvet Mittens made from sandpaper all depilated hair at the surface of the skin, but were expensive and likely to lead to skin irritation and scabbing.[24] Since tweezing hairs individually frequently proved too time consuming for densely covered areas, modified shoemaker's waxes were used to rip off large patches of enmeshed hair in a single motion. Such waxes, however, were challenging to obtain in bulk, difficult to apply, and painful to experience.[25]

Patent depilatories remained widely available in the early twentieth century, ranging from ineffective peroxides through

irritating, foul-smelling sulfides to outright lethal thallium compounds.[26] One young woman, ulcerated and scarred by a sodium
sulfide depilatory, lamented, "[T]here was nothing to live for. The
mischief done to my face and arms will last forever. I wish I could
go to sleep and never wake up again."[27] One of the most popular—and deadly—of these products, the thallium acetate depilatory Koremlu, cost only thirty-five cents per jar to manufacture
but sold for between five and ten dollars per jar. Prior to the passage of the landmark Food, Drug, and Cosmetic Act in 1938
(pushed to the fore of congressional attention due in part to injuries from depilatories), and before claims against the firm finally
forced it into bankruptcy, thousands of Koremlu users were either
killed or permanently maimed by muscular atrophy, blindness, or
limb damage.[28] Even relatively benign packaged depilatories often caused significant discomfort during use. One physician, Dr.
H. L. Baer, speculated that the pain associated with patent depilatories was not limited to the location of hair removal but might
also be transmitted "along the branches of the facial nerve to the
teeth and the tongue," where metallic fillings and bridgework
may help "to conduct the nerve current of the pain." Baer advo-
cated the placement of a wooden barrier between the teeth of the
patient during chemical hair removal to interrupt "the transmission of this nerve current."[29]

Razors of various types could also be used to remove hair at
the skin's surface, with far less pain—if more blood—than many
other methods. Yet commentators routinely noted the distaste
women had for shaving themselves, given longstanding associations between blades and manliness, and women's concern that
repeated shaving actually accelerated hair growth. (Physical an-
thropologist Mildred Trotter's classic 1928 essay establishing that
shaving does not accelerate hair growth did little to allay wom-
en's concerns on that point.)[30] As a final method for the temporary removal of hair, at least one period specialist recommended
a procedure known as "punching." With this technique, a slender
cylindrical knife was jammed through the skin around the hair

shaft and immediately withdrawn, leaving a severed column of skin containing the hair-root. Punching was never a particularly popular method of hair removal.[31]

Each of these methods, however effective, provided only transient relief from troubling hair, since the follicle itself often remained intact and capable of further production. For a more lasting effect, the woman of means might try electrolysis, a technique developed by physicians in the late 1870s and diffused alongside the increasing availability of portable electric batteries.[32] In electrolysis, a slender needle charged by a galvanic battery was inserted directly into the hair shaft. The electrical circuit was then closed and a slight bubbling at the skin's surface was produced as both the hair root and surrounding tissues were blanched. The hair was then easily removed with "epilation forceps" (more commonly known as tweezers). Both galvanic electrolysis and a later sister technique, diathermy (practiced with alternating rather than direct current), were complicated, expensive procedures typically practiced outside the home by experienced specialists.[33] Unlike razors, waxes, or depilatories, diathermy and electrolysis involved both a separate, skilled operator and sophisticated, spark-snapping machinery. The techniques not only required meticulous attention and skill on the part of that operator but also extreme patience and tolerance for pain on the part of the client, particularly the client seeking to remove hair from a large area of skin. The needle recipient's level of commitment to the procedure—her "tolerance"—actually enabled the very operation of the electrical equipment: she completed the electrical circuit by grasping an electrode of the machine or dipping her fingers into a dish of water.[34] As one physician described the procedure,

> When the needle is inserted the patient is directed
> to touch the electrode. She naturally touches it first
> with the end of one finger, adding gradually another one, till all five fingers are in contact with

the handle, ready to grasp the handle with the full
palm, if necessary, thus controlling by her own action the degree of intensity of the current.[35]

In order to ensure the full intensity of the current and thus the full
efficacy of the treatment, electrolysis experts often recommended
anesthetizing the client. Several specialists suggested applying a
mixture of cocaine and lanolin on the area intended for treatment,
in order to help "harden" the woman to her task (figure 4.1).[36]

The limitations of these methods make it easier to understand
why so many women might leap at the prospect of removing
hair through prolonged exposure to radiation. First introduced
by professional physicians in the late 1890s, x-ray hair removal
offered several distinct advantages over other techniques. To begin, x-rays were undeniably effective at removing hair, as even
the staunchest critics grudgingly admitted.[37] More important,
the rays transcended the grubby physicality of all other existing
methods of hair removal. Appropriately named "x" by discoverer
Wilhem Conrad Roentgen in recognition of their enigmatic nature, the rays were alluringly imperceptible. Gone were the noxious smells of depilatories, the root-ripping pain of hot waxes,
and the frightful appearance of multiple electrified needles. In
one popular chain of commercial hair removal salons, Albert C.
Geyser's Tricho system, clients were seated before a large ma-
hogany box containing the x-ray equipment.[38] A metal applicator
the shape and size of the area to be treated was adjusted to the
box's small front window, and the turning of a switch started
the operation. The x-ray equipment itself was visible to users
only through a small window in the front of the machine, and
the machine shut off automatically after the appropriate period
of exposure, usually three to four minutes.[39] The x-ray client
might hear the clanging, snapping sounds of electrical generation or detect an odd ozone smell, but the epilating rays themselves were clean, quiet, invisible, and mysterious (figure 4.2).

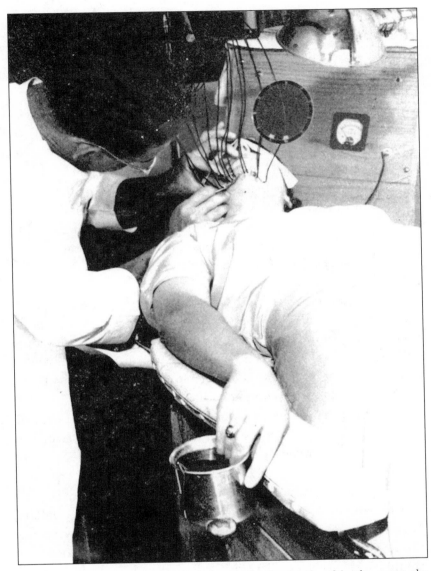

Figure 4.1. Multiple-needle electrolysis: by dipping her hand in the water, the woman being treated closes the electrical circuit, thereby controlling the intensity of the current and the relative speed (and pain) of the procedure. (From Bordeaux's *Superfluous Hair; Its Causes and Removal* [1942], reproduced courtesy of the American Medical Association.)

Needle experts expressed concern about precisely these qualities. Enclosing information on leasing options she had received from an x-ray salesperson, Cleveland-based electrologist Mary P. Searles wrote to the American Medical Association in Chicago for an informed second opinion on the new machine in 1925:

> For twenty-seven years I have removed superfluous hair by the electric needle & this prospect of doing away with the hard work necessary for the completion of a bearded face is indeed to be heralded with joy; however, I must know more about it before using one. I was very much interested, but since seeing how the sweat glands are dessicated [sic] in the enclosed pictures, I am dubious.[40]

Asserting that the lofty promises of the x-ray method seemed "ridiculous," another needle specialist wondered, "If this preparation could penetrate deep enough to kill the papilla [the large structure at the base of the hair follicle] what would prevent it from destroying all the adjacent tissue[?] Surely it couldn't be selective enough to just kill the papillae."[41]

Other beauty specialists were less worried about the physiological effects of the x-ray than about the threat of economic displacement heralded by the new machine. Electrologists accustomed to lucrative self-employment were alarmed by the prospect of prolonged financial indenture to a conglomerate such as Tricho, which required an initial fee of three thousand dollars, followed by ten years of 10 percent royalties.[42] Moreover, since the machine required no painstaking needle manipulation, any would-be beauty specialist with sufficient capital to hang out a shingle could operate it. One Oregon-based electrologist with twenty years' experience, Mrs. Jennie Stedman Farrell, wrote to the AMA to remark on the "prohibitive" cost of the advertised machine, and to express concern for the future of her occupation—the sole means of "living for myself and children."[43]

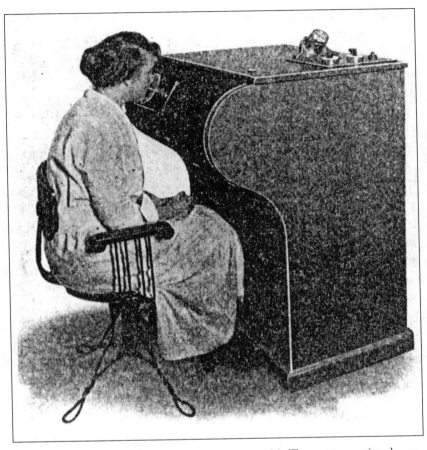

Figure 4.2. A hair-removing x-ray in use, circa 1925. (From a promotional pamphlet for a Detroit "Tricho" salon, courtesy of the American Medical Association.)

But most beauty specialists were not well positioned to reject the new ray. Geographically isolated in independent salons, economically dependent on a specialized method of hair removal, and then lacking the organization provided by a professional headquarters or publication, the specialists were hardly equipped to organize against the increasingly powerful Tricho corporation. Those who did contact medical professionals seeking help in preventing x-ray companies' "unfair and doubtful claims" of injury-free hair removal were repeatedly rebuffed.[44] At the same time, not all needle specialists were dragged by circumstances into x-ray work. While some embraced the x-ray in an attempt to out-compete other hair removal specialists, others appear to have adopted the machine in part because they sought personal access to toil-free, painless hair removal.[45]

Meanwhile, commercial salons seized the imperceptible nature of the rays as their primary selling point, eagerly perpetuating the promise of effortless transformation available with the x-ray. As one pamphlet assured, "The woman being treated absolutely does not feel, hear, or see the action of the ray."[46] Or, as a number of advertisements summarized the experience, "Nothing but a ray of light touches you."[47] The gentle new light would banish not only hair, the promotions further argued, but also the sticky, smelly, time-consuming labor once required for its removal. Hand tools such as tweezers and sandpaper were described as rudimentary, "Antiquated Methods," vestiges of a painful, tiresome past happily superseded.[48] One Boston newspaper advertisement urged prospective clients to think of the "joy of freedom from depilatories or razors" possible with the x-ray.[49] The theme of women's emancipation from routine, messy work was reiterated in a pamphlet from a Tricho salon in Detroit, which concluded simply, "It is no longer necessary for any woman to resort to the old makeshifts, since science has shown the perfect way."[50]

THE RAY'S IMPERCEPTIBILITY augmented a crucial aspect of its popularity: its association with "science." Like countless other businesses in the early twentieth century, hair removal salons learned that references to "science" both piqued customers' interest and provided the enterprise with an aura of legitimacy.[51] Appropriating this aura, salon operators made frequent references to the "scientific" methods and equipment used in their establishments, and to the "scientifically sound principles" on which their hair removal process was based. Yet the salons' references to science were not simply spurious: x-ray hair removal actually sprang from late-nineteenth-century physical research.

The hair-removing properties of x-rays were discovered accidentally by two Vanderbilt University researchers in 1896, within weeks of Roentgen's first public announcement of the "new kind of light."[52] In March of that year, Professor John Daniel and Dr. William L. Dudley were asked to locate a bullet in the head of a wounded child. As Professor Daniel later recalled the chain of events, Dudley, "with his characteristic devotion to the cause of science," agreed to lend himself to an experiment with skull x-rays. Twenty-one days after Dudley's head had been exposed for an hour with the tube placed a half-inch from his scalp, Daniel reported that all hair had fallen out from the area held closest to the tube.[53] News of the researcher's new bald spot spurred substantial "editorial merriment," as historians Ruth Brecher and Edward Brecher put it. "[T]here were even suggestions in the newspapers and technical journals that the X rays might render daily shaving obsolete."[54]

Soon after these "merry" speculations, professional physicians began to experiment with the x-ray in the treatment of hypertrichosis. In 1898, two Viennese dermatologists, Eduard Schiff and Leopold Freund, published the first good results of this medical therapy.[55] On the heels of their success, scores of dermatologists, roentgenologists, and other physicians in both Europe and North America adopted the effective new treatment.[56] By 1910, one specialist declared that the "electric needle, formerly so prevalent, but tedious and painful in operation, has largely given way to the X-rays."[57]

In fact, medical use of the electric needle never did give way to x-ray hair removal. Some European and North American physicians continued to use x-rays well into the 1920s to remove hair from skin intended for grafts or on skin affected by ringworm, but most U.S. physicians had grown reluctant to use the x-ray for other hair removal even before the First World War.[58] American physicians' abandonment of x-ray hair removal stemmed partly from their increasing recognition of radiation risk, as the passage of time provided further evidence of the latent effects of x-ray exposure.[59] Yet scientists, technicians, and physicians had grown wary of radiation "burns" prior to widespread experimentation with x-ray hair removal, and their support for the technique continued even as they witnessed the destruction wrought on the bodies of x-ray "martyrs."[60] It would be difficult, therefore, to attribute physicians' increasing reluctance to treat superfluous hair with x-rays solely to their sudden recognition of the effects of radiation on human tissue.

The eventual decline of medical x-ray hair removal reflected not only growing awareness of radiation risk but also physicians' unwillingness to apply the prestigious new ray to the treatment of body hair. Definitions of excessive hairiness remained maddeningly fluid, and the intractable ambiguity of the disease's diagnosis moved hypertrichosis to the contested border between "cosmetic" and "medical" concerns. Although medical practitioners readily conceded that body hair was a matter of intense concern to many women, hypertrichosis remained in the margins of professional therapeutics, the country cousin of more stately concerns such as cancer and tuberculosis.

The x-ray, on the other hand, enjoyed unquestionable sovereignty as one of medicine's crowning achievements. Abraham Flexner's 1910 report on American medical education, which lambasted the inadequate training and lax regulation evident at most of the nation's 155 medical schools, ushered in a wave of reform. In the wake of Flexner's report, some American physicians grasped for new ways to shore up their professional authority. For these post-Flexner physicians, the x-ray played a crucial role not only in medical diagnostics and therapeutics but also in enhancing the status of the medical profession itself. As a result, physicians grew increasingly reluctant to use the x-ray, a symbolically and materially potent therapy, on a problem that hovered on the fringes of professional respectability.[61]

Seeking to preserve the scientific clout of radiation therapy, many physicians endeavored to restrict its application by pressuring their colleagues to resist hairy patients' requests for x-ray therapy.

One practitioner urged his fellows to resist the natural temptation to comply with patients' eagerness to employ x-radiation, since their growth was a "cosmetic defect" rather than a "serious disease."[62] As another physician summarized, "It is not customary to shoot at sparrows with cannon-balls. Why, if we treat a hairy surface of the face of a fair lady, for instance, resort to means as powerful as those we employ in carcinoma?"[63] Through such admonitions, x-ray experts cast visible hair as "a purely cosmetic defect," superfluous to the proper domain of medical therapeutics.[64]

As professional physicians backed away from x-ray hair removal in the late 1910s, commercial practitioners were quick to fulfill demand for the technique.[65] New commercial x-ray salons were opened not only by nonmedical beauty specialists but also by those physicians and scientists squeezed out of reputable medical societies, professional publications, and other systems of collegial recognition due to their continued interest in x-ray hair removal. These practitioners readily presented clients with respectable diplomas and refereed publications testifying to their professional credentials, and their salons bore titles that alluded to the technique's scientific origins ("Hamomar Institute," "Kern Laboratories," "Hirsutic Laboratories," etc.). Commercial practitioners, in other words, drew on the same scientific aura physicians were attempting to define, protect, and control by disavowing this application of the ray. As professional scientists and physicians sought to prohibit x-ray hair removal, they unintentionally bolstered the technique's scientific prestige. Its popularity soared, and hundreds of x-ray salons opened across the country over the course of the next three decades.

WHILE SALON OWNERS and managers promoted the x-ray as the most scientific method of hair removal available, they never actually defined the term: the ambiguity of "science" was perhaps its most marketable feature. Yet as loosely and broadly as science was defined in hair removal advertisements, it was quite systematically linked to a notion of progress. Whatever else science might have been, it was invariably and unceasingly advancing.[66] A brochure for the Virginia Laboratories of Baltimore emphasized the endless progress of science, noting that the thirty years of refinement of the x-ray that had elapsed since Roentgen's discovery "can be said to be but a mere few minutes of time in the slow but certain development of knowledge." The advancement of science was further naturalized by likening it to the maturation of an awkward youngster. As the Baltimore salon put it, "great discoveries often go without much attention for a time, but inevitably they come into their own."[67]

Just as salon advertisements linked science to a notion of inexorable progress, this progress was in turn linked to the "strange power" of the x-ray.[68] Science, accessible through the enigmatic new light, could now at last fulfill the "dream of faultless skin."[69] One 1933 brochure, paradoxically titled "Be Your True Self: We Will Tell You How," proclaimed, "Our MODERN SCIENTIFIC METHOD with filtered RAYS" is "not 'just another' hair remover" but the only one that can "banish" one's dark traces. As the brochure pledged, "It is only a step from the Shadow into the Sunshine."[70] Commercial hair removal salons routinely stressed the value of "smooth, white, velvety skin" in their advertisements, linking the eradication of hair to the eradication of "troubling" racial markers.[71] The enlightenment offered by scientific knowledge and the woman's own visible, physical "enlightenment" were further entangled in one salon's letter to a prospective client: "Thanks to the progress of science, no woman need now endure the torture and selfconsciousness which a physical blemish causes." As the letter continued, more ominously, "Whatever you do—wherever you go—you need to have your skin CLEARED from this dark shadow."[72] The inevitable progress of science, such ads suggest, eliminates all darkness in its path. Scientific advancement yields personal, physiological transformation (figure 4.3).

As a notion of scientific advancement was linked to somatic enlightenment, so too were both narratives linked to dreams of upward class mobility. Through plentiful photographs of plush

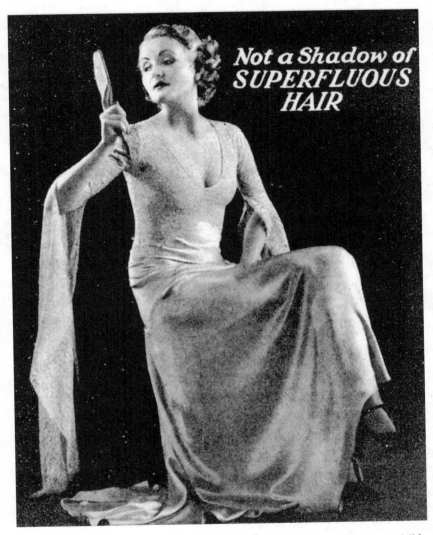

Figure 4.3. An advertisement for "Vi-Ro-Gen" of Pittsburgh, circa 1935: visible hair casts a dark shadow. (Courtesy of the American Medical Association.)

consultation rooms and sleek treatment rooms, promoters promised prospective clients a space unequaled in cleanliness and luxury.[73] Simply by stepping into the salon, claimed one testimonial, a woman was invited to experience the "padded carpets, the beautiful polychrome furniture, the soft shaded lights and dainty draperies, [and] . . . the quiet, restful atmosphere of . . . studious habits and refined tastes."[74] Many of the promotions made the economic importance of hair removal for women far more explicit. Prefaced by a line drawing of a well-dressed white couple approaching a cap-wearing attendant, a Chicago Marveau Laboratories ad demanded, "Can you afford to neglect your personal appearance any longer, in this age when it counts so much in social and economic advancement?"[75] Similarly underscoring the sexual (and hence economic) benefits of feminine hairlessness, the Dermic Laboratories of San Francisco and Los Angeles seconded this theme: "Freedom from Unwanted Hair Opens the Gates to Social Enjoyments That Are Forever Closed to Those So Afflicted" (figure 4.4). [76]

The salons knew their audience. Commercial x-ray salons targeted their promotions to urban, non-English-speaking populations, a fact noted by health officials seeking to warn the public about the practice.[77] Medical and legal records indicate that most x-ray clients were working women employed in low- or middle-income positions: telephone operators, secretaries, clerks, and so on. (While a few men used x-rays to remove hair from the face, ears, and neck, the vast majority of x-ray clients were women.)[78] Some former clients recalled receiving special group discounts at hair removal salons for bringing in large numbers of friends or coworkers.[79] Such discounts must have been attractive, for even in the midst of the worst economic depression the nation had seen, salons charged from five to thirty dollars each for a series of ten to forty treatments.[80] Even at those steep prices, tens of thousands—if not hundreds of thousands—of American women irradiated themselves in order to remove their hair.[81]

That thousands of working women struggled to save the vast sums necessary for these treatments points to the larger resonance

Long

Pickup By:
1/27/2020

.

.

.

.

.

.

Figure 4.4. A
Depression-era
advertisement
for "Dermic
Laboratories"
x-ray salons,
highlighting the
importance of
hairlessness to
class mobility.
(Courtesy of the
American Medical
Association.)

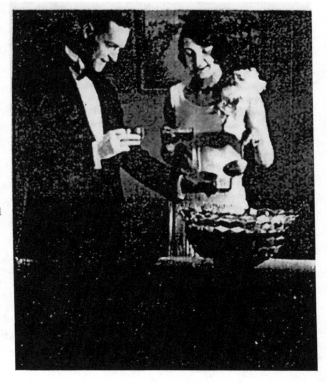

of the x-ray advertisements: the hope that personal, physical transformation might bring passage to new economic opportunities—to a world of "refined tastes." In the salons' promotions, a mist-enveloped "science" promised enlightenment at once somatic and social—with the x-ray providing the purchasable avenue to both kinds of development.

One can only speculate what role the advertisements' allusions to racial and class mobility played in the lives of the particular individuals who sought access to x-ray hair removal. Yet removing the "dark shadow" that barred access to the world of "social enjoyments" appears to have acquired fresh urgency during the interwar period, an era of increasingly restrictive U.S. immigration laws, widespread interest in eugenics, and increasingly desperate economic depression.[82] While women rarely spoke explicitly to questions of race in their letters about hair, they frequently connected their "affliction" to broader economic and social concerns. In one young woman's letter to the American Medical Association (AMA), for example, anxiety about her financial malaise and anxiety about her excessive hair flow into one another. Describing her frustration at the expense of x-ray treatments, the stenographer from Philadelphia concluded, "I am ever so anxious to find a cure for this affliction. This has been the cause of much unhappiness and actual sorrow to me."[83] Obviously troubled by the "considerable sum" she had already exhausted on x-ray hair removal, 25-year-old Anne Steiman expressed similar concerns from Brooklyn in 1933:

> I am working for quite a small salary now and I have saved every penny I possibly could[,] denying myself luxuries that all girls love toward trying to get rid of this unwanted hair, and believe me that saving this money was quite an effort as things at home are quite bad.

> But, I cannot go on as I am now, as I am miserable through a freak of nature and I have more than once thought of putting an end to my misery.[84]

Steiman and other young women of the nation's urban working poor could scarcely afford to ignore the possibility of economic uplift seemingly carried by a "complexion clear and fair."[85]

The few existing traces of women's direct responses to x-ray advertisements suggest that consumers were in fact impressed by the promotions' themes of advancement. When writing to beauty specialists and medical experts for advice on the x-ray, women often referred directly to advertisements that they had clipped and attached to their letters. One woman summarized the mood of these letters when writing to the AMA in 1931. Under the headline of a brochure from Philadelphia's Cosmique

Laboratories, Katherine Moore asked simply, "Doesn't this sound pretty good?"[86]

CLEARLY, THE X-RAY did sound good—not only to Katherine Moore and to Anne Steiman but also to the women who would, even after the technique was prohibited by state authorities, continue to try to sneak access to "back-alley" x-ray hair removal. As one agent with San Francisco's Homicide Detail reported in 1940, women had been seen entering an old rooming house at 126 Jackson Street "at various times of the day, subsequently leaving by . . . an alley at the rear of the building." After the women entered, a car would pull up "with a man carrying a case resembling . . . a doctor's kit. They would also enter the building for a short time, come out, and drive away."[87] At first sight, the medical kit, the furtive departures, and the decrepit building all signaled to the investigating agent the arrival of a "new abortion parlor."[88] The confusion is illuminating, for it demonstrates that for some women at least, hair removal was nothing less than a matter of life and death, pursued even as use of the x-ray was denounced in popular women's magazines and assailed by medical and legal authorities.[89] The act of "removing roots" appears to have held more than one meaning.

These meanings would change with the passage of time. By the late 1940s, the practice of x-ray hair removal had largely—though not completely—vanished. The demise of the practice could be explained in various ways. On the broadest level, one might take into account shifting commitments to ideals of whiteness. Particularly after the atrocities of the Nazi eugenic program, white Americans were forced to reexamine their malignant veneration of racial purity.[90] The reevaluation of radiation risk in the aftermath of the bombing of Hiroshima and Nagasaki further tarnished the appeal of commercial x-ray salons.[91]

While such major events abetted the decline of x-ray hair removal, the end of the practice ultimately stemmed from persistent, local activism. Clients themselves were at the forefront of this agitation, filing lawsuits and pressing regulatory officials and professional organizations for stronger action against x-ray salons. One Ohioan wrote to several agencies in 1931, trying to discern why Tricho salons were allowed to remain in operation. "I am just wondering what the U.S. Public Health Dept. is for, if not to safeguard the health of the citizens of the country, especially when asked specifically about something like this."[92] Responding to clients' complaints, various local and national Better Business Bureaus, local and state Departments of Health, Boards of Medical Examiners, women's magazine editors, and law enforcement agents attacked x-ray hair removal on multiple fronts throughout the 1930s. Some physicians lobbied for the revision of existing medical practice acts, which had overlooked the unlicensed use of electrical devices in the treatment of superfluous hair, while others swayed x-ray manufacturers to arrest production of commercial hair removal equipment altogether.[93] Local Better Business Bureaus pressured daily papers to refuse advertisements for x-ray hair removal, while metropolitan health officials used radio announcements to warn nonliterate consumers of the dangers of the practice.[94] The increasing prominence of severely disfigured or dying x-ray clients and their retributive claims against salon owners and workers must have also impacted the popularity of the procedure.[95] Articles lambasting the potentially lethal practice had been appearing regularly in medical journals and popular magazines since the early 1920s, and became more graphic with the passage of time, detailing gruesome cases of scarring, ulceration, cancer, and death. Some x-ray clients were so upset by the atrophy and other effects of radiation poisoning, particularly if their hairiness had been only "mild" in the first place, that they responded with attempts of suicide.[96] By 1940, after more than forty years of continual practice, x-ray hair removal had been driven out of the formal sector of the American economy, surviving primarily in surreptitious venues like the old rooming house at 126 Jackson.[97]

Yet even while coming to terms with their scarred and twisted bodies, many former x-ray clients continued to express hope for the special, personal promise of scientific progress. This promise is captured in the 1954 words of a former Tricho client (reproduced as in the original letter):

> The treatments were supposed to have been guaranteed, but within the last few year's "white spots" have appeared on my chin. This has been very heart breaking to me especially when on one's face.
> I have been wondering if ther might possibly be some new medical discovery which might help me. There are so many wonderful things happening these day's.[98]

Such faith in "new discoveries" would persist, as Americans' campaign against body hair adopted fresh tactics.

[5]

GLANDULAR TROUBLE

Sex Hormones and Deviant Hair Growth

IN 1946, THE *Science News Letter*, an American publication designed to convey breaking discoveries to the wider public, reported a novel transplant operation involving a young woman "of the bearded lady type." According to the two physicians who treated her, "overactive adrenal glands" had given the young woman an abundance of facial hair, and the woman had become "depressed" over her appearance. The two physicians persuaded the distraught patient to have her adrenal gland surgically removed, in order to slow the hair growth.

The extracted gland was then transplanted to a young woman with Addison's disease, a chronic adrenal condition manifested in this case by stomach trouble, depression, and darkening of the skin. Fourteen months after the transplant operation, the Addison's patient had been cured of her complaints. In contrast, the young woman who had donated the adrenal gland experienced unforeseen complications. Contrary to the doctors' previous experience with such surgeries, the patient's mental condition deteriorated after the gland was extracted, to the point that she began to suffer hallucinations. With additional psychiatric treatment, the patient was said to have recovered eventually—"left with only slight hairiness of her face."[1]

Such interest in the effects of glands on hair growth marked a consequential change in perceptions of human variation. Nineteenth- and early-twentieth-century assessments of hair, while plagued by problems of classification, tended to presume a fundamental divergence between the sexes: one might be a man or a woman but not both. Although comparative anatomists believed that amounts and types of hairs varied from species to species and from race to race, they did not hesitate to divide the sexes into two dimorphic categories. In contrast, explanations of hairiness based on glands and their various "internal secretions" presented sexual difference in more relative and mutable terms. By the time the *Science News Letter* reported on the experimental gland transplant in 1946, biochemists had detected "feminine" hormones in men and "masculine" hormones in women. Rather than approaching males and females as fundamentally distinct physical types, experts began to attend to the *"ratio* of maleness and femaleness in a single organism"—ratios that might be tweaked through specific interventions.[2]

In the course of that rethinking of maleness and femaleness, the locus of medical and scientific concern with hair shifted as well. Where natural philosophers from Jefferson to Darwin concentrated on comparative studies of the male beard, once hair distribution was linked to the glands, expert attention swung toward women. With the spread of endocrinology, women's "excessive" body hair increasingly was attributed to "an excess of androgens."[3] Efforts to manage such hormonal excess led to new pharmacological treatments. The availability of such systemic interventions, however, only aggravated the dilemma of determining exactly how serious hairiness needed to be to merit treatment.[4]

THE MANIPULATION OF ovaries and testes to influence appearance and behavior has a rich history. Aristotle discussed the extraction of sow ovaries in order to enhance the amount and quality of their meat; female camels used for military transport in the ancient world were spayed to abolish their estrus cycles.[5] Yet only in the nineteenth century did investigators begin to explore how gonadal manipulation—alteration of the ovaries and testes—affected the rest of the body. In 1855, French physiologist Claude

Bernard gave the name "internal secretions" to these still-mysterious forces, assuming like other physiologists of the time that their influence on the organism must work through the nervous system.[6] To learn more, Bernard and other physicians and physiologists tested the results of various transplantations and surgical excisions. As early as 1872, Atlanta physician Robert Battey, former surgeon to the Confederate Army, began advocating oophorectomy, the removal of ovaries, for an array of women's diseases. The ovaries that Battey removed were not themselves thought to be diseased; rather, he sought to induce premature menopause as a way to relieve diffuse symptoms of "nervousness." Over subsequent decades "Battey's operation" was performed on thousands of women in the United States, England, and Germany.[7]

Further experiments with glands proliferated after a set of trials conducted by the French physiologist Charles-Edouard Brown-Séquard. As a 72-year-old man facing the diminishments of age, Brown-Séquard injected himself with fluids concocted from the crushed testicles of guinea pigs and dogs. He attributed the renewal of vigor he experienced via this self-medication to some potent factor in the male gonad.[8] Although his discovery was derided by many colleagues (who apparently found the association with testicles too titillating), publication of his findings triggered a rush of therapeutic experiments in the 1890s.[9] Rudimentary gland extracts could be made as simply as brewed coffee: the animal gland, ground up and allowed to soak in grain alcohol or distilled water until coagulated, would be scooped into a semipermeable filter. As the liquid passed through the fine strainer of the filter and drained into a receiving jar, it took on some of the properties of the ground gland. The resulting liquid might then be further extracted with alcohol, acetone, or ether. Across the country, chemists, druggists, and kitchen experimenters tested various animal tissues in this way, including material obtained from human testes, ovaries, and placenta.[10]

Without formal regulation in place governing the testing and marketing of such extracts, the experimental drugs were soon applied to people.[11] Not long after Brown-Séquard's initial publication of his good fortune with ground testicles, a Parisian midwife self-administered a liquid made from crushed and filtered guinea pig ovaries, and an American physician soon began treating women with a similar brew.[12] Although physicians and physiologists often complained of being mocked for their study of gonadal extracts, the use of such drugs flourished.[13] Within months, newspapers and popular magazines were filled with advertisements for preparations made from animal glands, sold under names such as Ovarine, Ovaridine, Ovogenine, Oophorin, Biovar, and Spermine.[14]

Americans were soon ingesting a wide array of such glandular preparations: "minced fresh sow's ovaries taken in a sandwich, desiccated ovarian substance in powders or tablets, extracts made with water, glycerine, or alcohol."[15] The race to bring new preparations to market required huge amounts of animal material: mounds of ovaries or testicles were required to extract a single dram of secretory fluid. Thousands of tons of animal material— cow, sheep, horse, pig, dog, rabbit, guinea pig, mouse, and rat—

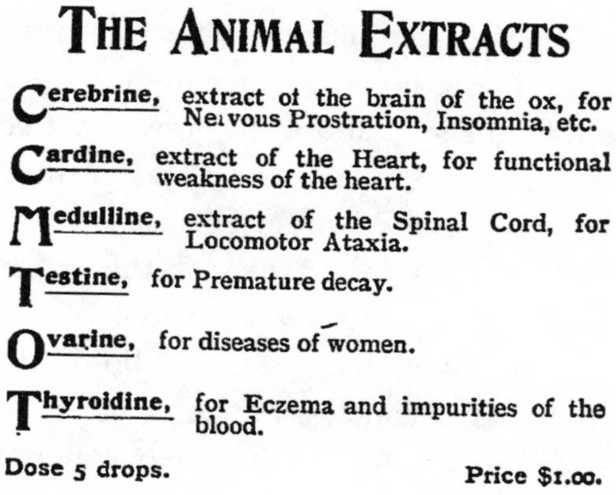

THE ANIMAL EXTRACTS

Cerebrine, extract of the brain of the ox, for Nervous Prostration, Insomnia, etc.

Cardine, extract of the Heart, for functional weakness of the heart.

Medulline, extract of the Spinal Cord, for Locomotor Ataxia.

Testine, for Premature decay.

Ovarine, for diseases of women.

Thyroidine, for Eczema and impurities of the blood.

Dose 5 drops.   **Price $1.00.**

Figure 5.1. One of the many late-nineteenth-century medicinal extracts, made from animal glands, used to curtail the growth of body hair. (Advertisement from *The Watchman* [1895].)

were ground into extractable pulp. Early experimenters recalled shuttling from packing plant to packing plant to obtain the requisite bodies.[16] Competition for the lucrative market in glandular therapies for women was particularly fierce. According to Robert Frank, a gynecologist at the Mount Sinai Hospital in New York, "the subject has attracted innumerable workers who are elbowing and jostling each other and jockeying for position," all rushing to develop preparations to relieve "the ills from which women suffer."[17]

DISTINGUISHING THE INFLUENCES of particular glands turned out to be difficult. Over the closing years of the nineteenth century, experimental anatomists, gynecologists, chemists, and physiologists all struggled to isolate specific agents of influence from glands, and to develop assays that could trace the production of those agents to specific groups of cells.[18] By the turn of the century, it occurred to the British physiologists William Bayliss and Ernest Starling that the glands' mysterious effects might be chemical in nature, transported through the body by the bloodstream rather than via the nervous system as previously supposed. On the advice of a colleague, in 1905 Starling termed these chemicals "hormones" (from the Greek "to excite" or "to set in motion"), likening their communicative function to that of a telegraph system.[19] By the 1920s, experimenters had defined the major glands in this system: pituitary, thyroid, adrenals, ovaries, and testes. By 1929, "female" sex steroids had been isolated from the urine of pregnant women; by 1931, "male" sex hormones had been isolated from the urine of men.[20]

In these early decades of chemical research, most experimenters assumed that female sex hormones existed only in people identified as women, and that male sex hormones existed only in people identified as men. Yet already by 1921, the alleged sexual specificity of sex hormones was being called into question: men's bodies, it seemed, also secreted "female" hormones," and women's secreted "male" hormones.[21] The specificity of sex hormones was further challenged by new findings in the late 1920s and early 1930s, including observations that testes extracts could cause changes in vaginal cell structure, and that the urine of stallions appeared to be a stronger source of estrogen than the urine of nonpregnant mares and geldings.[22] Initially, endocrinologists struggled to make sense of such observations; some felt compelled to include statements in their results that the urine tested came from men "whose manliness could not be in doubt."[23]

By the late 1930s, however, the gonads and adrenals of both men and women came to be considered sources of "male" and "female" sex hormones. As one 1939 review concluded, the fact that "all males secrete estrogens and females androgens" is "now well established."[24] For gland experts, the distinction between men and women was no longer seen as absolute but as "a matter of relative quantities of particular chemicals."[25] Secondary sexual characteristics, in turn, became part of the "index" by which "the sex composition of a man or a woman" might be established.[26] "Maleness and femaleness are best understood," wrote Louis Berman, a medical doctor and an associate in biological chemistry at Columbia University, as "the expression of chemical influence stimulating or depressing the evolution of the various characters we recognize as belonging to the sexes."[27]

The study of sex hormones thus seemed to confirm, on a chemical level, the observations of earlier sexologists: a slippery continuum existed between male and female traits. As Berman proposed, "One may then logically expect all sorts of combinations of sex characters to occur, which as a matter of fact do occur, and are roughly included in the term 'sex intermediates.'"[28] Berman further suggested that relative differences might vary even over the course of a single life: "[A]t one period of an individual's life his chemistry will be feminine," while at another, "his chemistry will be masculine."[29] A textbook published in 1939 captured this vision of variability succinctly: "There is no such biological entity as sex."[30] Chemical understandings of sex moved the fluidity of masculinity and femininity to the fore.[31]

IN FOREGROUNDING THE hormonal character of sexual difference, endocrinology confronted the divergent conceptual framework presented by psychoanalysis. The two fields expanded more
or less contemporaneously in the United States: Sigmund Freud
first visited the country in 1909, four years after Starling coined
the term "hormone"; the founding of the American Psychopatho-
logical Association and the American Psychoanalytical Association roughly paralleled the professionalization of endocrinology;
A. A. Brill's English translations of Freud's works accelerated the
spread of psychoanalytic ideas even as Berman and others were
popularizing glandular perspectives.[32]

Like endocrinology, psychoanalysis shared late-nineteenth-
century sexology's fascination with the development of non-nor-
mative sexual traits, including both "pathological" patterns
of hair distribution and "deviant" attitudes toward body hair.
And, like those earlier experts, psychoanalysts viewed hair as
a window onto "disorders" in sexual development. But unlike
endocrinologists, psychoanalysts focused on the genital and
anal symbolism of hair, linking hair and "hair activities" (like
brushing and shaving) to displaced sexual conflict.[33] In his famous 1933 essay on femininity, Freud focused on pubic hair
when tracing feminine "vanity"— concern with physical appearance—to penis envy, a "compensation for their original
sexual inferiority." Women's unconscious efforts to conceal their
"genital deficiency," he argued, drove their primary contribution to history:

> It seems that women have made few contributions
> to the discoveries and inventions in the history of
> civilization; there is, however, one technique which
> they may have invented—that of plaiting and weav-
> ing. If that is so, we should be tempted to guess the
> unconscious motive for the achievement. Nature
> herself would seem to have given the model which
> this achievement imitates by causing the growth at

maturity of the pubic hair that conceals the genitals.
The step that remained to be taken lay in making the
threads adhere to one another, while on the body they
stick into the skin and are only matted together.[34]

Such unconscious, psychic explanations for beliefs about hair ran
counter to the glandular thesis, which instead attributed emotion
to the action of internal secretions. "[I]n the final analysis," summarized one gland proponent in 1921, we are "very much the expression of the activities of the endocrines."[35]

Which experts, endocrinologists or psychoanalysts, might be
best suited to the alleviation of sexual disorders, including those
disorders concerned with body hair?[36] Some tried to strike a balance between competing somatic and psychic perspectives. André
Tridon, for example, argued for the fundamental inextricability
of psychoanalytic and hormonal approaches, emphasizing the "re-
ciprocal influence exerted by the mind on the glands and by the
glands on the mind."[37] But psychoanalysis, caught up in the same
reorganization of professional medicine that tightened restrictions
on the x-ray, lost this particular battle.[38] Even relatively restrained
psychoanalytic perspectives, like Tridon's, did not blunt endocrinology's ascendance in American thinking about body hair. By
1920, clinicians were routinely positing causal links between glandular disturbances and "masculine" hair distribution in women,
and those causal links were reiterated in the American popular
press. Gland proponent Berman declared there to be no feature
of the human body more swayed by the internal secretions than
the "quality, texture, amount and distribution of the hair."[39] Other
popular books of the period similarly insisted that the "amount
and distribution of hair on our bodies" is controlled by the "hormones or internal secretions of these glands."[40] Such texts helped
popularize the idea that patterns of "masculine" hair growth on
women indicated an underlying endocrine disturbance, such as
diseased ovaries or overactive adrenal glands.[41]

Endocrinologists' influence on understandings of hairiness

was reflected in the introduction of a new diagnostic category: "hirsutism."[42] Where the nineteenth-century physicians who first identified hypertrichosis defined the condition largely in reference to "dog-faced boys" and uncommonly hairy family lineages, the twentieth-century disease of hirsutism was tied specifically to women.[43] As the 1922 edition of Dorland's medical dictionary explained, hirsutism is "[a]bnormal hairiness, especially in women."[44] Abnormal hairiness, moreover, was increasingly characterized as stemming from glandular trouble. One influential 1921 paper railed against the idea that unusually hairy women demonstrated some kind of evolutionary atavism, insisting instead that the growth resulted from subtle, internal hormonal deficiencies.[45] Another 1921 editorial in the *Journal of the American Medical Association* concluded that the "bearded lady" was now properly regarded as one of the more visible "victims" of "disordered endocrine glands."[46]

Despite the seeming specificity of "glandular" explanations, the challenge of distinguishing truly "abnormal" hair growth persisted with hirsutism as it had with diagnoses of hypertrichosis. Over time, medical journals grew thick with charts and graphs designed to help practitioners sort normal from abnormal hair growth.[47] The most influential by far was a scoring system put forth by David Ferriman and J. P. Gallwey in 1961. Still known and used as the "Ferriman-Gallwey Index," the method employs a scorecard for each patient, surveying eleven (subsequently reduced to nine) different sites of the body (upper lip, chin, chest, upper back, lower back, upper abdomen, lower abdomen, upper arms, and thighs), each rated from zero (no extensive terminal hair growth) to four (extensive terminal hair growth). The numbers are added to attain a final score (figure 5.2). Although experts employing the scale continued to dispute exactly what final tally should indicate hirsutism, the relative ease and affordability of the test compared to other tools of measurement—such methodically counting the individual hair shafts per square inch—elevated its use.[48]

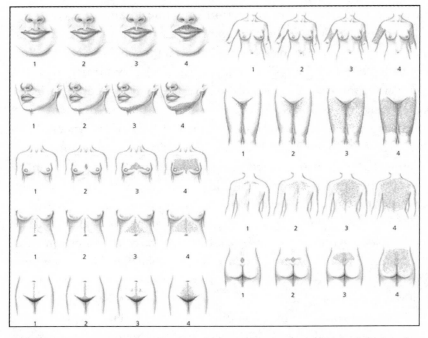

Figure 5.2. The Ferriman-Gallwey scale for evaluating excessive body hair, originally published in 1961. (Reproduced with permission of Endocrine Society.)

Such diagnostic scales, even the most quantitatively minded physicians realized, were precarious given shifting cultural attitudes towards women's body hair. As one physician lamented, "styles in eyebrows change as do those in gowns."[49] An endocrinologist at Harvard Medical School similarly explained that women suffering hairiness of the chest due to "pituitary deficiency" may be "prevented from wearing evening gowns."[50] To add to the trouble, the acceptable quantity of each type of hair varied as incessantly as class-stratified trends in clothing. The term "hirsutism," physician Howard T. Behrman concluded in the *Journal of the American Medical Association*, is "relative in that what might be considered excessive and unwanted depends upon the individual, the sex, and even the race." He explained, "[A] mustache is preferred by some men and unwanted by most women; yet, a light

growth on the upper lip of women is considered a sign of a lov-
ing nature in certain Latin countries and therefore is desirable
to a woman." Because hirsutism involves individual and collective "attitudes, styles, and beliefs," Behrman continued, "from a
medical standpoint . . . we are basically concerned with this problem when the hirsutism deviates sufficiently from the norm to
concern the person."[51] In other words, the level of patient distress
drove medical diagnosis—distress that was itself dependent on
mutable social norms.

AMONG THE MOST formative of those norms in the early twentieth century were intensifying injunctions against sexual inversion.[52] "Inversion," recall, was the elastic term used by sexologists
and other experts to refer to non-gender-normative behavior, deportment, fantasy, and appearance. Although experts remained
divided on whether hairiness revealed underlying sexual abnormality, many readily linked "inversion" to glandular trouble. Two
of the most influential sexologists of the period, Ellis and Hirsh-
feld, argued that all sexual development, including sexual inversion, "depended upon the glands of internal secretion."[53] The first
case discussed in a 1938 report on "Endocrine Aspects of Homosexuality" concerned a young man who "plucked his eyebrows,
colored his nails, and in other ways imitated women."[54] Alluding
to the homoerotic themes that gave rise to the word "lesbian,"
another report concluded that the "strange abnormalities" of the
ancient Greek poet Sappho of Lesbos probably resulted from "disturbance of her adrenal glands."[55] Others proposed that the links
between inversion and glands were "well established" and "past
dispute."[56]

With sexologists and endocrinologists connecting hairiness to
glands and glands to inversion, popular writers did not hesitate
to close the gap, attributing hairiness to sexual deviance directly.
As noted previously, correlations between hairiness and women's
sexual depravity have a long history in Western thought; lore associating hair with witchcraft, demonic possession, and wildness

dates back millennia.[57] Formal study of glands and hormones introduced fresh scientific terminology into aged prejudices. By the
mid-1930s, beauty manuals and advice columns, routinely attributing visible hairiness to an ineffable "glandular disturbance,"
were also hinting at its troubling sexual connotations.[58] In the first
English-language monograph on the topic, *Superfluous Hair and
Its Removal* (1938), Alfred Niemoeller devoted an entire chapter
to relations between "Superfluous Hair and the Glands." Citing
Havelock Ellis, Niemoeller declared that when hair distribution
on an adult woman "resembles the male's, it is frequently accompanied by some evidence of sexual inversion."[59] Another beauty
specialist, Delmar Emil Bourdeaux, made the point more bluntly:

> Excessively developed hair upon the body of the
> male suggests the brute. But in women the impli-
> cation is more disturbing still. The kind of superflu-
> ous hair with which women are usually afflicted is
> what we have come to think of as one of the normal
> secondary sexual characteristics of the male. The
> presence of such growths, especially facial growths,
> upon a woman suggests that she might perhaps be
> "queer."[60]

The collision of sexological and endocrinological attention to "excess" hair endowed such queer-baiting rhetoric with scientific authority, in all probability exacerbating cultural anxieties about
body hair and the dangers facing nonconforming individuals.
Visible hair, now thought to reflect "disturbances" in internal secretions, suggested stigmatized desires and behaviors.[61]

THE SUCCESS OF endocrinology not only altered American understandings of excessive hairiness; it also provided novel means
by which complications arising from "glandular derangement"
might be rectified.[62] Consistent with both expanding habits of
consumerism and principles of eugenics, management of the in-

dividual body came to be seen as a way to mold the larger social body—a way to eliminate degenerative vice of all kinds.[63] Modification was the name of the game. "Finally," wrote one Harvard physician in 1933, "the mental and emotional trends of the individual may also be determined in large measure by his hormones" and targeted accordingly.[64] The endocrine glands, "the origin of political extremism and antisocial behaviors," could be recalibrated through medical therapy.[65] Unlike psychoanalysis, endocrinology seemed to promise control of the individual "chemical machine," practical means for rendering humans—in Louis Berman's words—"less contemptible and more divine."[66]

Excessive hairiness in women, now generally depicted as stemming from an excess of male hormones, became one of the key targets of corrective "endocrine stimulation."[67] (As ever, just what constituted "excessive" hair remained flexible.) The overly "virile" woman might be feminized through modern surgical and chemical techniques.[68] Investigators undertook a range of trials involving surgical excisions, such as the experimental removal of the young woman's adrenal glands described in the *Science News Letter*, as well as injections of desoxycorticosterone acetate, adrenal cortical extract, and other hormone enhancements.[69] In the 1930s, pharmaceutical companies began producing chemically manufactured hormone preparations on a larger scale, opening possibilities for gland research and therapy.[70] With increasing production of steroid drugs, the development of new tools for determining the presence of androgen excretion in urine, plasma, and blood, and the advent of noninjectable hormone therapies (tablets and wafers) in the mid-1940s, glandular treatments blossomed.[71]

Historian David Serlin has traced growing interest in glandular intervention to a larger culture of "self-improvement" in twentieth-century America, in which medical care came to be seen as a purchasable amenity much like a household appliance or family car.[72] From existing letters, it appears that individuals troubled by hair did seek such medical reinvention. One expert, for instance, recalled the case of a young woman named Mae who sought help for a "face full of unsightly hair." Diagnosed with an "overactive gland," her "disturbance" eventually was "brought under control by her doctor."[73] In 1931 a woman from Urbana, Ohio, wrote several queries about appropriate techniques of hair removal, noting that she suffered superfluous hair "due to a glandular trouble, for which I am now under treatment."[74] The head of a boarding school in Dayton, Ohio, wondered whether a girl in his care, with visible hair around the upper lip and chin, might be the victim of glandular disturbance. The "deformity," he wrote to the American Medical Association, has "greatly affected her personality from a social point of view," and the "complex she suffers will not be removed, I think, until a permanent remedy is found." He sought the association's help in determining whether she might be aided by "glandular treatment."[75] The physician who replied to the headmaster noted that the AMA knew of "no medication aimed at glandular function which would accomplish a correction of this condition."[76]

Other physicians in the 1930s and 1940s were equally circumspect about gland therapy. "The medical profession is keenly aware of the fact that 'shotgun' mixtures of drugs have been grossly abused," wrote one endocrine expert. Moreover, "it is widely believed" that once the "primary endocrine defect" is recognized and treated, the "secondary abnormalities will thereby in turn be corrected." Yet because the physician's "endocrine tools" are "few and mostly dull," such corrections are rarely guaranteed.[77] In the absence of strict regulation, however, far less modest claims ran amok. One Chicago physician complained to an influential friend that his daughter, seeking hair removal, visited a commercial salon run by a man called Jacques L. Abbott. Abbott insisted that clients completely disrobe in order to receive "vibratory" treatments for the "'stimulation' of the 'sexual gland.'" Such a "scandalous" situation, the friend affirmed, was "intolerable."[78]

THE TENTATIVENESS EXPRESSED by medical experts in the 1930s and 1940s evaporated by the early 1950s, as researchers abandoned the challenging physical excision and insertion of glands or gland extracts in favor of oral drug therapy. If the suffering endured by hairy women seemed to most physicians undeserving of the risks associated with early surgeries or concoctions, hair reduction seemed a perfectly reasonable application for emerging hormonal therapies. Ethinyl estradiol or oestradiol was one of the first; within a decade its use was entrenched. Prednisone/progesterone treatment of hirsutism began in earnest in the early 1960s.[79] By the early 1970s, physicians were regularly prescribing two types of hormonal drugs to retard body hair: suppressive therapies designed to lower high plasma androgen levels, and anti-androgen therapies designed to counter the effect of androgens at the hair follicles. Two of the most commonly used of such pharmaceuticals, spironolactone (often marketed under the name Aldactone) and cyproterone acetate (often sold as Androcur), have since been distributed to millions of women as straightforward medical necessities, including to growing numbers of male-to-female transwomen.[80] Within thirty years of the experimental adrenalectomy described in the *Science News Letter*, glandular treatment had become standard medical practice. Treatment turned from symptomatic relief through shaving or electrolysis toward "systemic control of hirsutism."[81] Both physicians and patients sought to eradicate body hair through "pharmacological means."[82]

As with earlier chemical depilatories, the advent of new therapies sparked debate over the relative weight of the suffering caused by "disease" and "cure." These debates were particularly pointed given the potential side effects of systemic hormone therapy: cancer, stroke, heart attack, and so on. Moreover, several of the drug combinations developed in the postwar period were found to *stimulate* hair growth—on the upper lip, the inside of the thighs, and elsewhere.[83] The adverse effects of prolonged drug regimens for hirsutism were particularly troublesome, one physician noted, given that most of the women seeking treatment were of child-bearing age.[84] Pregnancy apparently altered calculations of value.

Yet even as medical journals were filling with accounts of successful treatment of hirsutism with anti-androgens, a new prospect was emerging: that of abandoning hair removal altogether. "[A]lready," noted one prominent medical journal in 1976, "some younger women are leaving body hair alone. The reason may be current fashion, indolence, a respect for untouched nature, women'[s] lib, or some other individual attitude. Who can say what the custom will be ten years from now?"[85] More radical approaches to the problem of hair were on the horizon.

[6]

UNSHAVEN

"Arm-Pit Feminists" and Women's Liberation

IN THE SUMMER of 1972, as the United States sat mired in a deepening war in Vietnam and facing an acrimonious presidential election, the editors of *Ms.* magazine prepared their first regular issue for distribution. The issue included essays on the value of housework, lesbian love and sexuality, and the Equal Rights Amendment. Joining such concerns to the forthcoming national elections, the cover displayed the cartoon figure of a strident Wonder Woman alongside the caption "Peace and Justice in '72" (figure 6.1).

But it was not merely the magazine's pursuit of peace and justice that resonated with readers, nor its consideration of labor in the household, sex between women, or an equal rights mandate. It was a three-page essay sandwiched between those articles, titled "Body Hair: The Last Frontier." There, authors Harriet Lyons and Rebecca Rosenblatt described the idea that "a woman's underarm and leg hair are superfluous" as an "embodiment of our culture's preoccupation with keeping women in a kind of state of innocence, and denying their visceral selves." Some women, they continued, go so far as to shave their pubic hair, "thereby emulating the infantile sexlessness of a little girl." Hair removal was declared to be one more measure of the drudgery to which American women were unjustly subjected. Yet an "emerging feminist consciousness" promised to counter the inequity, revealing the social forces arrayed against looking and smelling "as we really are." As the authors concluded confidently, while "the hirsute woman is not yet an idea whose time has come . . . more and more individual women are risking those stares to affirm their natural femaleness. Eventually, this small but intimate tyranny will be resisted."[1]

Lyons and Rosenblatt were accurate in their sense that the time had not yet fully arrived for the hirsute woman. During the Republican national convention later that summer, the *Chicago Sun-Times* columnist Irving Wallace was walking along a Miami beach with reporter Walter Cronkite when Cronkite asked if he had seen "the new Women's Lib magazine." Wallace responded: "Yes, I read it—about body hair on women—how they should let hair grow on their legs." He continued, "I don't like it, but there are some good arguments for it, Walter." According to Wallace's recollection, Cronkite nodded and replied, "I guess there are, but I just can't get used to it."[2] Cronkite's dismay about unshaven women was shared by others.[3] A letter to the *New York Times* in 1973 decried "arm-pit Feminists, women whose involvement with the ethic of body hair has overpowered other considerations."[4] One Texas legislator was said to have referred to the twenty thousand people who attended the 1977 National Women's Conference in Houston as "hairy-legged zoo girls."[5]

Even self-identified feminists weren't sure they were ready to cross the body hair frontier. *Ms.* decided to publish the piece after it had been rejected by *Cosmopolitan*, but even the article's editor, Suzanne Levine, reportedly found the idea of allowing hair to grow "a little disgusting."[6] Betty Friedan soon began criticizing Gloria Steinem and other *Ms.* contributors for telling American women "they didn't have to bother to wear makeup or shave their legs." Friedan heaped scorn on *Ms.* for "titillating . . . with sermons about unshaven armpits and pubic hair," while she and others focused their sights on enhancing women's professional mobility.[7] For Friedan, her biographer explains, "hairiness" became convenient shorthand for "anti-man, anti-marriage, anti-motherhood pseudo-radicals"—an efficient way of referring to all those activists Friedan considered "outside the mainstream."[8]

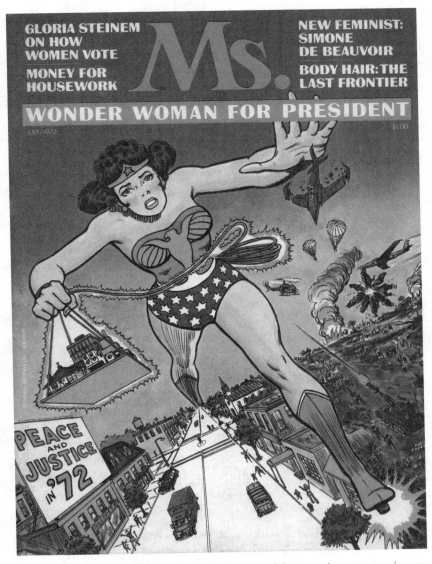

Figure 6.1. The cover of the first regular issue of *Ms.* magazine, announcing an essay on body hair. (Reprinted by permission of *Ms.* magazine, ©1972.)

What made hair such a ready surrogate for both proponents and critics of the social movement that came to be known as second-wave feminism? Why would the simple cessation of shaving be described, on the one hand, as a "titillating" diversion from more serious feminist concerns and, on the other, as dangerous political extremism, a sign of opposition to men, marriage, and motherhood? How did body hair come to be such a potent, conflicted symbol of women's political consciousness?[9]

Like blue jeans, bare feet, recreational drug use, and other elements of dress and deportment, body hair gained renewed symbolic resonance with the social change movements that emerged after the Second World War. No other element of countercultural style, however, developed such a lasting association with "feminism" as did visible leg or armpit hair.[10] Even a generation after the second wave, the American movie star Julia Roberts prompted international media frenzy by exposing a hairy armpit at a 1999 movie premiere. A major Canadian newspaper proposed that Roberts's unshaven armpit "was probably some feminist statement type thing rather than laziness," while the U.S.-based *Newsweek* suggested that a more fitting career for the actor might be "politics" or "teaching."[11] At the 2010 Golden Globes a decade later, the unshaven legs of award-winning actress Mo'Nique prompted a similar flurry of online and print commentary, much of it devoted to discerning her intended political "statement."[12] Americans' identification of feminism with body hair was still so well entrenched in the early twenty-first century that one review could sum up the entire, complex history of diverse U.S. women's movements with a single parenthetical allusion to "underarm hair."[13]

For both advocates and critics, unshaven armpits and legs served as a symbolic reminder of women's labor—in this case, the repetitive, expensive, and often invisible labor of maintaining hair-free flesh. The question of whether such efforts were a trivial nuisance (as Betty Friedan gruffly suggested) or the very embodiment of women's oppression (as Lyons and Rosenblatt argued) would shape discussions of women's bodily choices for decades to come. Women's hairy underarms and shins were transformed into badges of political consciousness, and the "hairy feminist" into an enduring cultural icon.

BEFORE ANY U.S. women could take up a call to stop shaving, however, they first had to be convinced to *start*, a shift that rested on several entwined technical and social developments. As noted previously, through most of the seventeenth, eighteenth, and nineteenth centuries, non-Native American women and men largely avoided self-shaving, due in no small part to the skill and care required to maintain a steel straight razor. That aversion slowly began to recede with the introduction of safety razors, which included a guard over the blade to inhibit inadvertent slicing. Described by French artisan Jean-Jacques Perret as early as 1770, the first safety razors were not brought to market until the late nineteenth century, where they enjoyed only modest success in the United States.[14] Although a marked improvement over "cut throat" razors, the blades on the hoe-shaped devices still required time-consuming honing and stropping. The more significant technical development was thus the 1903 introduction of the now-familiar T-shaped safety razor with double-edged, disposable blades. The blade, designed by King Camp Gillette, was brought to manufactured reality by William Emery Nickerson, an MIT-trained analytic chemist who had worked previously for an association of leather tanners. With Gillette's new razor, users were freed from the tedious labor of blade maintenance (figure 6.2).[15]

Shaving's appeal, particularly for women trained to feel shame about use of "masculine" tools, was further augmented by the introduction of private, indoor bathrooms. Prior to the development of public water systems and indoor household plumbing, obtaining the water needed for rinsing razor and skin was a back-breaking activity: water was gathered in buckets from ponds, streams, or water-hauling carts, pumped and hauled from wells, cisterns, and rain barrels. Bathing was an understandably rare event, even

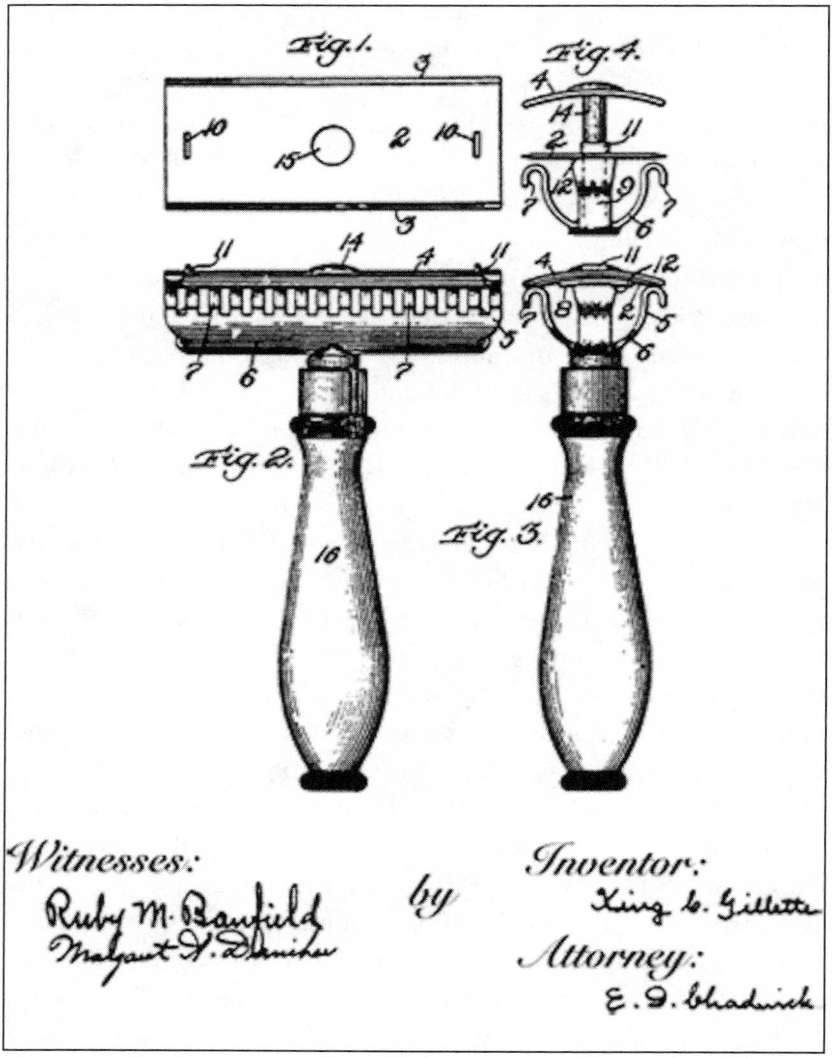

Figure 6.2. King C. Gillette's 1904 patent for a new safety razor, recorded by the United States Patent and Trademark Office.

for the affluent. Describing her first shower in 1798, Elizabeth Drinker, the famously beautiful wife of a wealthy Philadelphia merchant, noted that she had not been "wett all over at once, for 28 years past."[16] As urban populations grew, received approaches to water delivery and drainage became untenable. Driven by concerns about epidemic disease, major cities began developing municipal water supplies early in the nineteenth century; Philadelphia's pioneering water distribution system, constructed in response to recurrent outbreaks of yellow fever, began operation in 1801. Within a century of the nation's founding, most cities over ten thousand had at least some public water supply.[17] This shift did not mean that Americans had yet changed their daily habits. Bathing remained an irregular activity, even for those Americans wealthy enough to possess a fixed bathtub with piped-in water. For most, bodily washing remained tied to a bowl and pitcher set in an individual bedchamber, filled with water hauled by hand into the house. In 1880, five out of six Americans "were still washing with a pail and sponge."[18]

But as the nineteenth century drew to a close, perceptions and practices of bodily washing shifted. Immersed in a growing preoccupation with personal and societal cleanliness, bathing was transfigured from an elite affectation to a matter of personal and national health. The bathroom was described not only as a novel convenience but also as a bulwark against contagious disease.[19] Increasing numbers of municipalities installed public water mains and sewers, and pushed their growing immigrant populations to adopt new norms. "Every child," the New York State Department of Health declared in 1914, "should have one tub bath daily."[20] The urban poor, whose tenements did not yet include space or plumbing for middle-class amenities, generally relied on municipal bathhouses for washing; the rural poor continued to haul water by bucket as before.[21] Maintaining a separate, private area of the home for bodily washing—a "bathroom"—became a way to mark class status, and middle-class Americans strove to attain the luxury. Beginning in the 1870s, factory assembly significantly dropped the price of plain and enameled cast iron tubs and other standard bathroom fixtures. By 1908, consumers perusing the Sears catalogue could find a choice of three complete bathroom sets—tub, sink and toilet—for prices ranging from $33.90 to $51.10, all shipped ready to be connected to household plumbing.[22] Many of these bathrooms contained mirrors, also made newly affordable by mass production, which allowed fresh scrutiny of one's hair growth.[23] New home construction and urban planning reflected Americans' changing expectations, and support for public bathhouses declined accordingly. By the mid-1930s, nearly all of the apartments in New York City had private baths or showers.[24] More and more energy, water, metal, and stone were required simply to sustain what was considered "normal, ordinary, and necessary."[25]

More to the point, the advent of the bathroom facilitated shaving's passage from the public barber shop to the private space of the home. Where shaving previously relied on the help of paid or unpaid assistants, razors could now be used, safely and discreetly, in a room equipped with running water, drainage for effluvia, and a well-lit mirror. Shaving, formerly conducted by men on men in public, male spaces, moved into a sequestered room dedicated to maintenance of the body, where it could be practiced in unobserved solitude. The labors of hair removal were newly individualized and concealed.

The privatization of shaving in the United States continued with the nation's entry to the First World War. As King Camp Gillette's biographer notes, "the raising of mass armies, with millions of men in uniform and under strict discipline," offered unprecedented opportunities for introducing men to self-shaving.[26] Shaving appeared advantageous to military leaders for several reasons: not only did beard removal help keep down lice and other vermin, but it also helped assure a close fit for the gas masks used in the trenches. By the time American soldiers joined the conflict in Europe, U.S. Army regulations required every soldier to possess a shaving device of some kind.[27]

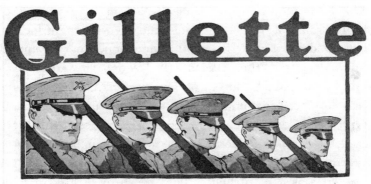

36   THE SATURDAY EVENING POST   *May 19, 1917*

Gillette

The Armies of the World Use the Gillette Safety Razor

WAR is the great test of any article of utility. The soldier's kit is reduced to actual necessities.

You can't imagine a soldier carrying 'round a strop and hone.

The Official Army Regulations of all Countries now call for a clean shave. And beyond all question the Gillette is the Razor of the Great War—of all the Armies, on all fronts.

Gillette Razors and Blades have gone abroad in a continuous stream of shipments from this Country—by thousands, by hundreds of thousands and by millions!

One recent shipment was 80,000 Razors and 600,000 dozen Blades.

They've gone by Atlantic Passenger Steamers—by Freight—by International Parcel Post. By first-class registered mail and they've gone as personal baggage with passengers. They've gone by Pacific Steamers to Japan and through Manchuria, then via the Trans-Siberian Railway to Russia.

Isn't there a lesson in this for every man in America who has not yet adopted the Gillette Shave?

We venture to say there is not a man living with a beard to shave but can shave better with a Gillette—if he will use it correctly.

If there is any man who is not enthusiastic over the Gillette it is probably because he has not caught the simple knack of using it.

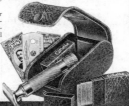

The Gillette is so efficient that men continually take advantage of it by cheating on the lather.

Be fair to the Gillette; soften the beard with a thick lather, well rubbed in, the same as you would with any other razor.

Insert a fresh blade, screw the handle down tight. Use a light, slanting angle-stroke. You will find the beard slips off almost like magic.

Now dash the face with cool water and pat dry with a soft towel.

There are thousands of young men just coming to shaving age. The Gillette will help them to form good habits—the saving of small sums that count up to big ones—the habit of getting started on time—of doing a thing perfectly in the quickest way, with the fewest motions.

Write for the New Gillette Catalogue. See the thirty styles of Gillette Safety Razors, $5 to $50. Gillette Dealers everywhere.

Milady Décolleté is the dainty little Gillette used by the well-groomed woman to keep the underarm white and smooth

If You Live in Canada—write the Gillette Safety Razor Company of Canada, Ltd., 73 St. Alexander St., Montreal, for Canadian Catalogue and Prices.

GILLETTE SAFETY RAZOR CO.
BOSTON, U. S. A.

NO STROPPING   NO HONING

Figure 6.3. A 1917 advertisement for the Gillette Safety Razor, stressing its place among the soldier's vital "necessities." (Courtesy of Matt Pisarcik, *RazorArchive. com.*)

The Gillette Safety Razor Company shrewdly anticipated this emerging market and began churning out special compact pocket razor and blade sets embossed with the insignia of the U.S. Navy and Army. They further allied their war effort with a new advertising campaign, trumpeting the shipment of "millions" of razors and blades to men fighting overseas. "You can't imagine a soldier carrying 'round a strop and hone,'" one advertisement for the disposable blades stated.[28] "[B]eyond all question," another 1917 advertisement declared, "the Gillette is the Razor of the Great War."[29] In less than two years, hundreds of thousands of American men were initiated into the custom of regular self-shaving (figure 6.3).[30]

Gillette was equally canny about bringing that military custom back to the home front. As the nation demobilized, the company ramped up its campaign. It opened a chain of luxuriously appointed stores, launched a fleet of shiny Franklin convertible cars marked with the company's logo, and sent out teams of young women to stage product demonstrations and address questions about shaving. By the time the company's patent ran out in November 1921, Gillette had helped acculturate "a whole generation of men from all classes . . . to the idea of the daily shave."[31] For American men, a freshly shaven face became "a normative cultural value."[32]

War also transformed women's relation to shaving, albeit in different ways. The Gillette Safety Razor Company introduced its first razor for women, the Milady Décolletée, in the midst of the European conflict. Small and curved to better fit the armpit, the razor was designed to supplement the sleeveless and sheer-sleeved fashions of the period. Yet increased pressure on women to remove their underarm hair did not translate simply or easily into greater comfort with the idea of shaving. Although depilatories remained messy, foul smelling, and—in the case of Koremlu—potentially lethal, many women continued to use them to avoid the masculine connotation of razors. Recognizing consumers' ongoing aversion to the concept, Gillette studiously avoided the term "shaving" and "blade" in advertisements for their carefully ornamented Milady Décolletée, referring instead to modern kinds of "toilet accessories."[33] Yet once American men returned from the war with established shaving habits of their own, women in their households might use men's razors sur-

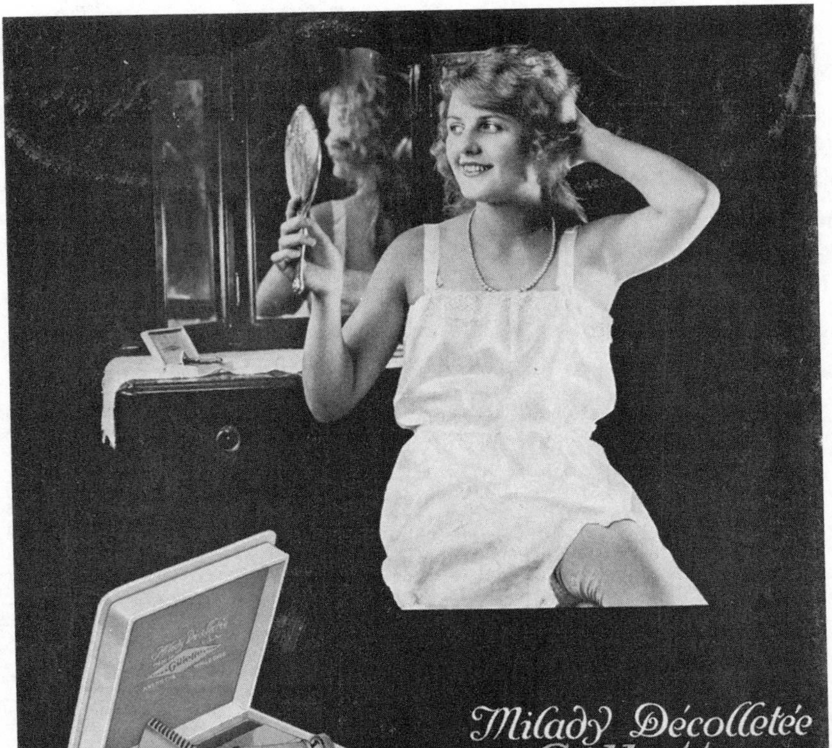

Figure 6.4. Early Gillette advertising copy for a women's safety razor, which carefully avoids reference to "shaving" or "blade." (Courtesy of Matt Pisarcik, *RazorArchive.com*.)

reptitiously, bypassing the stigma and hassle of purchasing their own tools for shaving. That women regularly swiped the razors of their husbands, fathers, and brothers is suggested by one magazine's reflection on the rise of razors designed for women: "The practice of 'razor-napping' has long been a source of mild marital and familial discord, and the greater availability of women's razors may even be a boon to family harmony."[54]

American women's gradual conversion to shaving reached a turning point with the production shortages brought on by the nation's entry into World War II. Animus against visibly hairy lower legs had been in place for two decades, but most women adhered to the social norm by wearing thick, hair-concealing stockings when appearing in public. As both nylon (a synthetic fiber developed by Du Pont) and silk were commandeered for military uses, stockings fell into increasingly short supply.[55] Two months after the Japanese attack on Pearl Harbor, Du Pont converted its nylon production—90 percent of which had been devoted to stockings—to military applications, even as raw silk imports from Japan ceased.[56] While England prioritized hosieries as an "essential" element of civilian life, the U.S. War Production Board sharply curtailed stocking manufacture: within a single year beginning in September 1941, production of all-silk hosiery declined 99.1 percent and all-nylon hosiery by 97.1 percent.[57] The resulting stocking shortage led to a dramatic rise in consumption of "liquid stockings," tinted compounds designed to create the illusion of fabric for women reluctant to appear bare legged. Sold as powders, lotions, and creams, leg cosmetics were applied with the fingers or an applicator pad—a process that could take anywhere from five to fifteen minutes a day, with additional time for drying and buffing. Sometimes paired with decals or penciled-in lines to create the illusion of a stocking seam on the back of the leg, "seam" and liquid stocking together cost only a fraction of the price of either silk or nylon stockings: where stockings cost on average about thirty dollars per month, effective liquid stockings were only about a penny per day, with a package of twelve "seam" decals running an extra twenty-five cents.[58]

The cosmetics only worked, though, when the legs were freshly stripped of hair. As consumer magazines emphasized, "The best liquid stockings available will deceive no one unless the legs are smooth and free of hair or stubble. Leg makeup will mat or cake on the hairs and make detours round the stubble and give a streaky appearance."[39] Shaving was essential for a "professional appearance" with the paints.[40] Despite the laboriousness of the process of shaving, painting, and striping, leg cosmetics gained popularity over the early 1940s, moving from fad to custom in a matter of months.[41] Several writers predicted that the use of the cosmetics would "go right on flourishing" even once silk and nylon stockings became available: "[T]hey're cheap, they're cool, [and] they never sag at knees and ankles."[42]

Wartime shortages, however, eventually caught up with the lotions, too. Beginning in 1942, the War Production Board, the agency appointed by President Roosevelt to convert the nation's industrial capacities to making munitions and other military equipment, set limits on cosmetics manufacturing along with other production deemed "nonessential." The popularity of leg cosmetics took another hit with the imposition of federal cosmetic taxes as high as 20 percent. By 1945, *Consumer Reports* noted that sales in leg make-up had leveled off, as more and more white women decided that it was cheaper and simpler to shave, "get a good coat of tan and let it go at that."[43] Regular shaving gained appeal, and continued to expand in the immediate postwar years, as women who adopted the practice in their teens and twenties passed the habit on to their daughters. By 1964, surveys indicated that 98 percent of all American women aged fifteen to forty-four were routinely shaving their legs.[44]

These changing social norms were eagerly supplied by a growing "personal care" industry, which expanded with the larger postwar boom in manufacturing. A hoe-shaped safety razor with replaceable cartridge (rather than simply replaceable blades) was introduced in 1970, and a hoe-shaped discardable razor—which required no maintenance or replacement of parts whatsoever—

was brought to market five years later. Both tools, priced to be marketed as disposable, relied on novel methods of plastic injection molding. And both tools carried with them the ecological implications of the postwar plastics industry, including consumption of petroleum and other composite materials, carbon emissions from production and incineration, and generation of solid waste, urban litter, and marine pollution. As historian of design Thomas Hine has observed, a "disposable world" had been created—a world that activists began to challenge.[45]

HOW DID A custom as widespread as leg shaving—widely adopted by 1945 and practiced by nearly all premenopausal American women by the mid-1960s—come to be targeted by proponents of "women's liberation"? Part of the answer lies in hair's prominent role in other emerging movements for social change: as a noticeable and relatively malleable physical feature, hair became a ready medium for communicating altered political consciousness. For advocates of Black Power and Black Nationalism, revised treatment of head hair became a vital element of resistance to racist perceptions of beauty. Rejecting pressed or chemically straightened hair was a way to "decolonize" the maligned black body, to directly challenge color-caste hierarchies that framed blackness as ugly or monstrous.[46] Unprocessed hairstyles, referred to as "natural," provided a visible bulwark against Eurocentric standards of appearance.[47]

Hair also acquired heightened political significance within escalating youth protests against the ongoing American war in Vietnam. Increasing numbers of male high school students, particularly white students, grew their hair long, infuriating some parents and school officials. Although no public consensus emerged on the meanings of young white men's uncut hair, for some observers the "hippie" style symbolized a "refusal to embrace the rationality, moderation, security, and orderliness that modern society expected from the best and the brightest of its young."[48] In 1967, the musical *Hair* picked up on this generational conflict. Structured around one young man's struggle to decide whether to comply with the draft, the musical merged seemingly superficial questions of dress and hairstyle with larger questions about violence, liberty, and social duty. The theater-going public embraced the show, and its commercial success further solidified the associations between hair and contemporary social movements.[49]

As head hair was acquiring new political connotations, women were identifying and articulating new political demands. Middle-class white women's increased participation in the paid labor force during World War II reconfigured their expectations of economic equity, as did the expansion of access to colleges and universities after the war. Growing disillusionment with sexism in the burgeoning civil rights, free speech, and antiwar movements further propelled some activists to enunciate distinctive positions within opposition politics. Feminist activists involved in Asian American "yellow power" organizations, the Chicano *Movimiento*, and American Indian struggles for sovereignty similarly staked out progressive roles for women within their respective movements for change.[50]

Such political agitation, importantly, tended to focus on spheres formerly considered outside the realm of politics. Having gained many of the characteristic political and economic rights of self-governance (the rights to control their own earnings, to hold and transfer property, to enter into contracts, and to vote), liberal and radical women (and men) increasingly turned their attention to matters long held to be "private." Sexual relations, the nature of the family, housework, and medical care all came to be treated as rife with persistent inequity. As activist Charlotte Bunch argued, "there is no private domain of a person's life that is not political and there is no political issue that is not ultimately personal. The old barriers have fallen."[51] Reflecting on her domestic life after reading Friedan's 1962 *Feminine Mystique*, one Atlanta housewife spoke for many when she declared that for too long she had "voluntarily enslaved" herself within the home.[52] Routinely echoing this language of enslavement, the dominant voices of second-wave feminism—white, middle-class— sought to extend "liberation" to the "prison" of the private home, the "subtle bondage" of sexual relations, the tyrannies of caring labor, and other domains.

WOMEN'S BODIES WERE at the center of these calls for liberation. For more than a century, achieving bodily self-determination had been a key objective of struggles for women's equality, evident in nineteenth-century radical Ezra Heywood's assertion of "Woman's Natural Right to ownership of and control over her own body-self."[53] In the 1960s and 1970s, support for rights to self-ownership and bodily control animated many of the activities of women's liberation, as reflected in the title of one of the era's most widely read books, *Our Bodies, Ourselves*. The idea that women should "take control of their own bodies" informed approaches to issues ranging from violence against women to participation in organized sports. Freedom and equality, activists proposed, resided in increasing command over one's "own" body.[54]

Body hair readily denoted this evolving regard for self-ownership and self-determination. The treatment of armpit, facial, or leg hair, like the changing head hair styles of antiwar hippies and Black Nationalists, provided women's liberationists with a malleable and visible symbol of their commitment to the "natural," unconfined body. Simply by ceasing shaving, advocates of women's rights might quickly establish their identification with larger social movements. Indeed, the representational power of hair was especially potent for women's rights advocates, given that routine removal of body hair so readily evoked the myriad other elements of so-called women's work that second-wave feminists were beginning to question. The shaving of women's pubic hair before hospital births, for instance, became one of several routine obstetrical interventions challenged by advocates of "natural" childbirth, along with mandatory episiotomies, the use of enemas, and the immediate withdrawal of newborns from their mothers.[55] As women gained new rights to determine their sexual and reproductive lives through landmark court cases such as *Eisenstadt v. Baird*, *Roe v. Wade*, and *Doe v. Bolton* (which together established the rights to use contraception and to terminate pregnancy within the first trimester), they also began to fight constraints on other kinds of bodily expression, such as prohibitions on cross-dressing.[56] Routine shaving—setting "your flesh . . . on fire"—was targeted as one among many "barbarous rituals" associated with womanhood in America.[57] In this context, body hair provided a convenient stand-in for larger disputes over which elements of the self were (or should be) subject to the woman's individual control. As expressed by one Seattle-based YMCA employee, fired for refusing to remove "excessive hair growth" from her chin, "If God gave it to me, why should I have it off?"[58]

Many of the white feminists who took up body hair as a badge of heightened political consciousness were not particularly reflective about the legacies of racial injustice invested in attitudes toward body hair. "The fact is," Germaine Greer comfortably declared in 1970, "that some men are hairy and some are not; some women are hairy and some are not. Different races have different patterns of hair distribution." "Some darkskinned Caucasian women have abundant growth of dark hair on their thighs, calves, arms and even cheeks," she continued, while "[t]hat most virile of creatures, the buck Negro, has very little body hair at all."[59] In their feature article in *Ms.*, Lyons and Rosenblatt noted, without critique, that visible body hair marked one not as a member of dominant American culture but as a "dirty foreigner."[60] They exemplified the point with an anecdote meant to shock the magazine's readers: "A young woman involved in a bicycle accident was asked by a New York policeman examining her injured, unshaven leg, 'You're not Puerto Rican, are you?'"[61] The iconic "hairy-legged feminist" was implicitly or explicitly coded as white and U.S. born.

Equally important, the racially coded rhetoric of women's liberation was easily converted to revenue-generating ends. Over the course of the 1970s, individual bodily control, rather than adherence to norms of hygiene or health, became the dominant theme of popular representations of hair removal. That ideal of bodily control, moreover, supported new trends in hair *removal* as readily as new trends in hair growth. Mainstream U.S. women's magazines shifted from describing body hair as "superfluous" or "excessive," as defined according to some abstract medical standard, toward describing hair as personally "unwanted." Through titles such as "Six Ways to Get Rid of Unwanted Hair," "Removing Unwanted Hair Permanently, Not a Do-It-Yourself Job," "Hair You Don't Want," and "Hair That You Can Do Without," magazines stressed the hope of liberation through consumption— specifically, the choice to purchase and use specific hair removal products.[62]

A GENERATION LATER, hair removal remained a flashpoint for battles over women's sexual and political freedom. In 1998, for instance, an Equal Employment Opportunity Commission appellate judge awarded compensatory back pay with interest and benefits for the harassment endured when a driving instructor referred to the appellant's "big old hairy legs" during a driving test.[63] Far more than their predecessors in the 1970s, however, "third wave" feminist activists began to oppose the corporate capitalism that encouraged the conflation of choice and consumerism. Spoken word artist Alix Olson expressed such opposition in her 2001 "Armpit Hair [Mammally Factual]":

> *Well, I want to go to Europe, the land of Brave and Free*
> *Where it's considered natural for girls to be hairy.*
> *Where Gillette don't make a profit off of*
>   *keeping womyn busy*
> *As pleasers with their shavers*
> *and their razors and their tweezers.*[64]

A group of self-described "radical cheerleaders" similarly challenged the nexus of corporate profit and hair removal, calling on the "goddess" as they rallied against a brand-name depilatory:

gals say no to nair!

we like our armpit hair!

if the goddess meant 4 our legs to B bare

she wouldn'TA put hair down there!

so gals say no to nair!

gals say no to nair!

FUCK YER FASCIST BEAUTY STANDARDS![65]

Other commentators proposed that resistance to hair removal was itself a dangerous sign. As references to "bearded terrorists" began proliferating in mainstream media after the attacks of September 11, 2001, some commentators began linking hairy-legged women to violent radicalism.[66] In 2006, a leaked version of a promotional pamphlet from the National Rifle Association—ominously

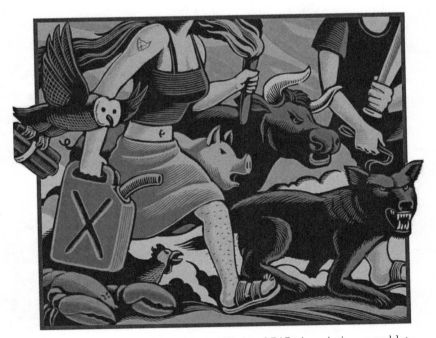

Figure 6.5. An image from the 2006 National Rifle Association pamphlet, *Freedom in Peril*, focused on the unshaven legs of the "Animal Rights Terrorist."

titled *Freedom in Peril*—used an illustration of a woman's striding, visibly hairy legs to represent the distinctive threat of "Animal Rights Terrorists." Even as some online commentators questioned whether the leaked document might be a hoax, they also highlighted the image of the hairy-legged terrorist as particularly compelling.[67] Visible body hair on women signaled political extremism (figure 6.5).

Thus pushed from opposite ends of the political spectrum, women's body hair became an indelible symbol of women's political consciousness, one that equated "freedom" with the ability to manage one's own individual bodily capacities.[68] Paradoxically, such individual choice was elevated as a virtue even as mundane bodily care was ever more entwined in vast, opaque networks of labor and resources.

[7]

"CLEANING THE BASEMENT"

Labor, Pornography, and Brazilian Waxing

RESIDUAL DEBATE OVER the political meanings of hairy armpits or shins was largely swept to the side with the rise of so-called Brazilian waxing in the early 2000s. A "Brazilian" entails removing all or nearly all hair from the genital area, including the vulva, anus, and perineum (figure 7.1). Adoption of the practice soared after Carrie Bradshaw, the main character of the popular HBO television series, *Sex and the City*, described the procedure in a 2000 episode.[1] Within a decade, some estimates suggested that one in five American women under the age of twenty-five were maintaining consistent, complete removal of their genital hair. A large survey published in 2010 indicated that at least a quarter of all women aged eighteen to sixty-eight had completely removed their genital hair within the previous month.[2] Some men, too, began adopting the practice; of the majority of American men who reported regularly waxing or shaving body hair from below the neck, a portion were opting for the complete genital depilation variously known as "Brozilians," "guyzilians," "manzilians," or, simply, "back, crack, and sack" waxes.[3]

PARTICULARLY GIVEN THE physical pain associated with total genital waxing (the pioneering Carrie Bradshaw described her procedure as a "mugging"), the practice took off with astonishing speed. Even as Americans expressed concern about visible hair on

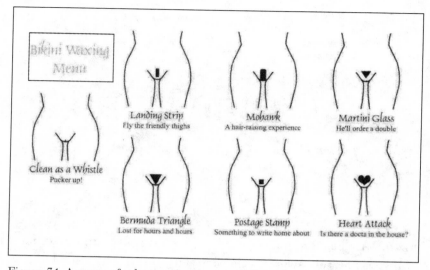

Figure 7.1. A menu of salon waxing options, frequently reposted on the Web in the early 2010s. This version appeared in an April 2013 blog.

women's arms, underarms, and lower legs in the first half of the twentieth century, few appeared to have worried much about pubic hair. Prior to the close of the Second World War, the rare references to genital hair removal in medical or popular literatures typically accompany reports of pathology.[4] Middle-class American women did not begin publicly displaying their pubic hair until the introduction of the bikini in 1946; even then, pubic hair removal was not widely practiced. Through most of the twentieth century, pubic hair appears to have been considered sexually appealing, and genital depilation remained uncommon.[5] As late as 1971, an informal survey of university students found that while 98 percent regularly shaved their armpits, very few shaved or shaped their pubic hair in any way. More than three-quarters of the women surveyed at that time described pubic hair as "a powerful weapon in their sexual armory."[6] By the late 2000s, however, clinicians were reporting it to be "unusual" to treat any woman under the age of thirty who still had her pubic hair, and perfectly routine to see eleven- or twelve-year-old girls with "pubic razor stubble."[7] Within a single generation, female pubic hair had been rendered superfluous.

Even as total genital depilation was becoming more widespread (so to speak), observers were expressing concern about what the practice suggested about contemporary American politics, particularly the status of women. One Minneapolis newspaper columnist lamented that "[t]hirty . . . years ago" women "across the United States . . . carried picket signs advocating free love and the ERA [Equal Rights Amendment]," while that "generation's granddaughters," in contrast, "are getting breast implants and Brazilian waxes."[8] Similar themes of liberation gone awry resounded through scholarly and popular writings, with genital waxing summoned as a sign of American women's deeper political confusion. Ariel Levy's best-selling 2005 book, *Female Chauvinist Pigs*, opened by mocking those young women who viewed themselves as *"empowered* enough" to remove all their pubic hair.[9] The habitual "shaving and waxing . . . [of] women's genitals," another writer concurred the same year, amounts to an act of "self-mutilation," one for which the "whole notion of consent must be thrown into doubt."[10] In 2007, a reader responding to an online article about genital waxing echoed that critique:

> We may think in the west that we are free—but we
> have been brought up constantly under the pressure
> of advertising—in the form of peer pressure and
> other social normalisation. . . . Yes women may of-
> fer up their bits voluntarily rather than at the end of
> a barrel of a gun, but the desire to do so comes from
> our enthrallment to consumerism.[11]

"[W]e are slaves," the commentator concluded, "yet we think we are free."[12] Converting such perspectives into public policy, in 2009 the New Jersey State Board of Cosmetology proposed an outright ban on genital waxing, after two women in that state were hospitalized with severe postwax infections.[13]

The proposed ban on Brazilians was quickly squelched by the practice's many advocates. To its proponents, the popularity of total depilation hardly indicated American women's enslavement but rather their exceptional political freedom. Genital waxing was not "the battle that liberation lost," as critics complained, but instead an emblem of American women's uncommon powers of bodily self-determination.[14] To some observers, *opposition* to hair removal appeared as the real tyranny—an illegitimate constraint on a woman's inherent right to own her own body and to dispose of its unwanted biological products as she saw fit. "[F]eminism wants you to be whoever you are," opined Jennifer Baumgardner and Amy Richards in 2000's *Manifesta*, even if you "shave, pluck, *and* wax."[15] When an essay posted online compared the penchant for waxing found in affluent industrialized nations to the kinds of ritual genital cutting commonly associated with northeast African communities, a reader indignantly insisted that "there is a difference" between the female genital modification practiced in the United States and U.K. and that practiced in "other cultures," a difference that hinged on "will": "Whereas in the west people are doing it willingly and with full knowledge of dangers involved, the female vaginal mutilation [in other locales] is done under pressure, if not force by the families and the cultures."[16] Advocates and critics of depilation were thus generally dedicated to similar ideals of self-determination; the two differed only in how "free"—and foolish—they perceived American women's choices to be.

As we have seen, principles of bodily self-determination have informed American discussions of women's hair removal since the liberation movements of the 1970s. There are, however, other stories to be told about the efflorescence of Brazilian waxing, beyond the wisdom or error of particular choices. Crucial in this regard are the wider conditions that made routine pubic waxing widely accessible in the first place—a global circulation of goods, people, and capital often ignored in favor of praise or condemnation of individual women's decisions to wax. Even the language currently used in reference to genital depilation hints at these larger conditions. The term "Brazilian" itself (frequently used in the United States as a noun rather than an adjective) is an American neologism. Scholar Magdala Peixoto Labre points out that the so-called Brazilian is not practiced by most women in Brazil; when the complete removal of pubic hair is conducted, it is referred to by the more technical name of "tricotomia." Labre traces the circulation of the name "Brazilian" to the influence of J. Sisters, a salon in New York operated by seven Brazilian siblings whose names all begin with the letter J.[17]

This chapter describes the ascendance of what might be better called "American" waxing, moving from the influence of mainstream and pornographic media to the manufacturing of wax products themselves. These symbolic and material developments unfolded within broader political and economic shifts—global changes generating new configurations of labor, capital, suffering, and freedom.

WHEN ASKED ABOUT pubic hair removal, most American women tend to describe their efforts as a form of "self-enhancement"—a way to feel cleaner and more attractive. While some report opting to remove hair in accordance with their sexual partners' preferences (and specifically, to encourage their partners to perform oral sex), most instead stress themes of hygiene and sexual desirability.[18] Beginning in the early 2000s, popular media reinforced these themes, tying complete genital waxing to celebrity glamour.[19] Gwyneth Paltrow's relatively early adoption of total genital waxing was widely reported to have "changed her life"; Kirstie Alley described the feeling as "like a baby's butt, only all over."[20] The enhancement provided by complete genital waxing also became a plot element in popular film: in the 2006 comedy *The Break-Up*, the newly single female protagonist, played by Jennifer Aniston, goes "full Telly Savalas" and walks naked through the condominium she still shares with her ex in order to tease and entice him.

Male hair removal, too, was promoted and understood as a form of self-enhancement, as signaled by the coining of the term "manscaping," generally traced to a 2003 episode of the television program *Queer Eye for the Straight Guy*. Much of the attention to male waxing in mainstream popular culture focused on chests and backs, as in the actor Steve Carrell's expletive-laced chest wax in the 2005 Universal Studios comedy, *The 40-Year-Old Virgin* (a scene that spawned dozens of imitative, homemade videos on YouTube). But the advent of male fashion trends, such as low-riding jeans, that focused on the pubic area and buttocks also drew scrutiny to previously covered areas of the body. Some commentators further speculated that both gay and straight men, influenced by pornography, began removing their pubic hair as a way to make their penises appear longer.[21] Male privates, too, were now public, and were subject to elective enhancement.

THE CULTURAL UNVEILING of genitalia in popular film, television, and online forums stemmed from the steadily increasing commercialization of erotic images over the twentieth century, and particularly the liberalization of censorship laws beginning in the late 1960s.[22] In *Redrup v. New York* (1967), the U.S. Supreme Court affirmed the right of consenting adults in the United States to possess and read written fiction with ostensibly obscene subjects without interference from the state; in *Stanley v. Georgia* (1969), the U.S. Supreme Court ruled that possession of other "obscene materials" in the private home was not subject to government regulation. Four years later, the Court's decision in *Miller v. California* effectively rendered "pornography" legally meaningless at the federal level, by allowing individual states to set "community standards" of decency. With a few important exceptions (such as child pornography, which the Court held enjoyed no constitutional protection under the First Amendment), individual states could henceforth determine their own laws regarding pornography.[23] Although in some jurisdictions the effect of these changes was to curtail access to pornographic material, the more general trend was to render films and publications more genitally explicit. Entrepreneurs opted to risk fines or jail time for showing more overt material in exchange for larger sales.[24]

Pubic hair was a key element of this strategy. The first widely circulated pornographic film to show pubic hair, Michelangelo Antonioni's *Blow Up*, was released in 1966; in August 1969, the American dancer and actress Paula Kelly became the first model in a *Playboy* pictorial to display plainly visible pubic hair.[25] Spying the lucrative potential of these efforts, theater owners began pushing films with full female nudity concentrated on the genitals—so-called beaver films. The Roxie Cinema in San Francisco ran a steady program of titles such as *Beaver Picnic*, *Beavers at Sea*, *Beavers in Bloom*, *Eager Beavers Demanding Their Rights*, and *Beaver Protest*. The popularity of more explicit films spurred development of smaller venues, which could evade community zoning regulations because they had too few seats to qualify as "theaters." As pornographic theaters and arcades proliferated, directors and producers began experimenting with still more graphic content: spread labia ("split beavers"), manipulation of the genitals ("action beavers"), and the addition of sound ("talking beavers").[26]

As the name implies, "beaver" films focused on female pubic hair.[27] But as pornographic producers continually sought to up the ante on graphic content to remain competitive, they also branched into new areas. In 1975, *Hustler* magazine published photographs of very young models without visible pubic hair under the headline "Adolescent Fantasy." The feature provoked "enthusiastic responses" from male readers and organized outrage from feminists: the political action group Women Against Pornography coalesced the following year.[28] To critics, the popularity of the *Hustler* spread affirmed Harriet Lyons and Rebecca Rosenblatt's contention that American hair removal practices demonstrated a "preoccupation" with the "infantile sexlessness" of little girls.[29] Whatever led producers of pornographic content to move toward hairless female models, move they did: content analyses confirm a sharp decline in visible pubic hair on nude centerfold models, as well as a tendency to minimize the appearance of the labia majora and minora.[30] One retired porn actress recalled of her work in the 1980s, "I posed with a full bush. No one in adult entertainment shaved back then. Now everyone does."[31]

How influential were such pornographic images on ordinary people's grooming habits? Studies suggest that consumption of porn does in fact affect hair removal practices. The prevalence of bare genitals in pornographic material, one review concludes, leads "to a perception that bare genitals are more erotic."[32] And, by the turn of the twenty-first century, most American women as well as men reported having viewed pornography. Aestheticians report not only that many men ask their wives and girlfriends to imitate the looks displayed by porn actresses and models, but also that women often request their first full genital waxes as special "surprises" for their partners before weddings, anniversaries, or Valentine's Day.[33]

WHILE THE APPEAL of hairless genitals owes much to changing pornographic and mainstream media, the rapid diffusion of total genital depilation would not have been possible without access to affordable, effective tools of hair removal. Waxing fit this bill well. One of the oldest techniques of hair removal still in wide use, waxing entails the application of a heated compound of natural and/or synthetic materials to unwanted hair. Once the hair adheres to the cooling and hardening goo, it is yanked out, either with the application of supplemental cloth strips or, if the wax is of the "hard" variety, without. Evidence of the similar use of resins for this purpose dates to ancient Egypt.[34] More recently, sixteenth-century English memoirs discuss the use of shoemaker's waxes to combat "hirsute intruder[s]," while nineteenth-century medical treatises recommend combinations such as "Plaister[s] made of very dry pitch" pulled off with leather.[35] Yet the use of waxes to remove hair was relatively rare in the United States before the twentieth century, limited to the occasional use of the melted tip of a candle or stick of sealing wax to remove stray whiskers. As distaste for hair growth on arms, armpits, and lower legs accelerated after World War I, interest in waxes increased. Innovative entrepreneurs began manufacturing and distributing hair removing waxes through the federal postal system, recruiting customers through advertisements placed in popular women's magazines. Under names that generally played on received Orientalist tropes (e.g., "Moorish Haire Removing Wax") or the prestige of modern science ("the Lanzette Method"), companies repackaged common sealing waxes as glamorous products. Some, like the wildly popular "Zip" wax, combined a wax hair remover with a sulfide depilatory cream.[36]

Most of today's waxes bear only passing resemblance to those earlier compounds. Although homemade pastes made from some sticky combination of sugar, honey, lemon, and water remain in use, popular commercial waxes are now generally based on a sludgy consequence of industrialized petroleum refining called "slack wax," supplied from small batch distributers located near major oil refineries.[37] Slack wax, a combination of oil and water, is heated, mixed with solvents, and then chilled; as it cools, more refined wax crystallizes out. Wax specifications such as melting point, penetration, and oil content may be adjusted by controlling the temperature and rate of cooling and by adding solvents. The wax is then further refined, passing through a bed of clay to remove color and through a vacuum stripping tower to remove odor. These refined waxes are blended together to generate particular properties, and further blended with polymers or other petroleum by-products to generate additional flexibility or glossiness.[38] Anticipating increasing pressure on the availability of petroleum derivatives, natural wax producers are already gearing up for increased exports of cosmetic-grade wax (figure 7.2).[39]

The conversion of petroleum waste into valuable by-product has been expedited by the current regulatory climate, which separates regulated "drugs" and largely unregulated "cosmetics." In the United States, hair removing waxes—like other compounds

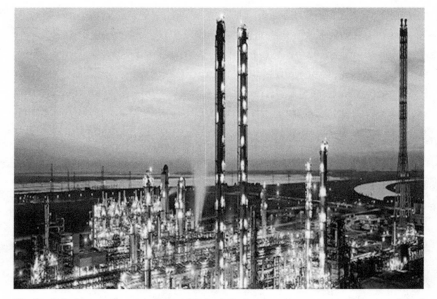

Figure 7.2. A petroleum refinery. Today's hair-removing waxes often consist of by-products of global oil production.

intended to be applied to the surface of the skin, such as lipsticks and nail polishes—fall under the regulatory directives of the "cosmetics" section of the Food, Drug, and Cosmetic Act of 1938. This classification means that both hair removing waxes and their myriad ingredients are released from mandatory premarket testing procedures.[40] (In contrast, the depilation of nonhuman mammals in U.S.-based meat and leather production is subject to relatively intensive federal and state surveillance.) In the absence of mandatory federal regulation of technologies used "merely" for "cleansing, beautifying, or promoting attractiveness," brands proliferate: literally thousands of different hair removing waxes are now available to consumers. The leading manufacturer in the United States, GiGi Wax, is a trademark of American International Industries, founded in 1971 and now one of the largest privately held beauty companies in the country.[41] The excrescences of transnational oil production have been turned into gold.

THAT CONVERSION WOULD not have been possible without the swift and massive shift in capital from crumbling manufacturing sectors into producer and consumer services after 1970. Already by 1977 private and public service employment accounted for two-thirds of all jobs in the United States, with novel health and beauty services comprising a significant slice of the sector.[42] According to the U.S. Census Bureau, gross receipts from "personal care services" between 1997 and 2002 grew at a rate of 42 percent.[43] Rapid expansion in American cosmetic products and services was mirrored in other parts of the affluent world, as capital investment in industrial manufacturing similarly shifted to service sectors. By 2003, the skin care segment of the global cosmetics industry alone was generating more than $24 billion annually, according to analysts at Goldman Sachs. Established conglomerates such as Unilever or Procter & Gamble began devoting significant resources to acquiring and consolidating their share of the beauty business, as when the luxury goods holding company LVMH purchased the fledgling cosmetic lines Hard Candy and Urban Decay.[44]

As markets for such consumer services segmented and matured over the closing decades of the twentieth century, investors and service providers struggled to identify and cultivate new fields of income growth: hair removal provided a lucrative answer to that problem (recall that American women who wax spend an average of twenty-three thousand dollars on hair removal over the course of a lifetime). Some previously untapped populations—teenagers, men, and high-income older women—were encouraged to adopt novel practices of depilation.[45] Some longstanding habits of hair removal, such as care of the eyebrows, were given fresh emphasis; one search reveals a 232 percent increase in references to "eyebrow waxing" in English-language publications between 1984 and 2000.[46] Along with waxing, other labor-intensive methods of hair removal were promoted. Among the most popular was threading (also known as *bande abru* or *khite*), in which the skilled practitioner pulls a doubled, twisted thread over the unwanted hair.[47]

At the same time, previously ignored regions of body hair—such as hair on the back, anus, or perineum—were newly targeted for modification. Waxing is often the technique of choice for such regions, since it is far more efficient and cost-effective for removing hair from irregular patches of skin than plucking, threading, or electrolysis. It is for this reason that industrial poultry production often relies on hot wax for defeathering (figure 7.3).[48]

Each area of the body, in turn, might be managed iteratively. Because a Brazilian may be repeated every three to six weeks, a consumer might visit one salon this month and a second salon the next, depending on price, ease of purchase, and other factors, or to adopt one pattern of pubic topiary at one turn and another subsequently.[49] One could first try a design called a "Tiffany's Box," in which pubic hair is shaped, bleached, and dyed into the robin's-egg-blue square typical of the luxury jeweler's packaging; one could subsequently wax the skin bare

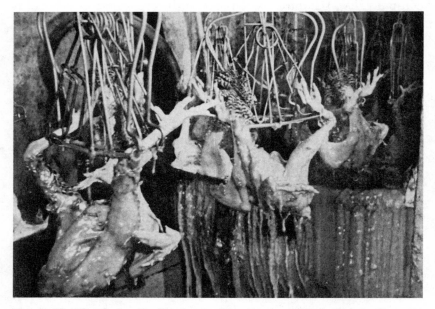

Figure 7.3. "Depilating Poultry by the Wax Process," photograph by Berenice Abbott. From Siegfried Giedion's *Mechanization Takes Command* (1948).

and add a heart-shaped pattern of glued-on crystals or feath-ers.[50] Rendering more and more hair "superfluous" and inces-santly modifiable in such a way provides recurrent sources of economic growth.[51]

SERVICE LABOR IS at the heart of that growth. Because it is fairly difficult to remove one's own hair from some of the regions of the body now targeted for cosmetic treatment—the anus, say—depilation usually requires the paid or unpaid labor of a skilled second person. Moreover, because that labor cannot be conducted remotely (as many other kinds of medical, educational, and fi-nancial services can be), it cannot be outsourced to workers in dis-tant locations. The service workers who perform the sticky work of genital waxing are tied to their client's bodily location. In this sense, genital waxing bears important similarities to the forms of service provision—housekeeping, child care, elder care—more typically studied by theorists of postindustrial labor.[52] The analogic relationship between hair removal and such labor was handily summarized by aesthetician Pegi Carnahan in 2003: "What makes a Brazilian a Brazilian," said Carnahan, "is when I 'clean the basement.'" At the time of that interview, Carnahan was cleaning at least five "basements" a day in a Seattle beauty salon.[53]

Just as with housework, sex work, and in-home dependent care, the tedious and inescapably manual labor of body waxing is subject to remarkably little legislative or professional oversight, whether practiced in salons or in homes. In the United States, each state crafts its own laws and statutes concerning sanitation, sterilization, and infection control, as well as those regulating the boundaries between medicine and cosmetology or between cosmetology and other nonmedical licensed specialties such as "aesthetics." Even where relatively strong laws and regulations do exist, there is little money for enforcement. The Enforcement Unit of the California Board of Barbering and Cosmetology, for example, employs only fifteen inspectors for the entire state.

Given overwork, boards generally only investigate salon workers once a complaint has been filed.[54]

And, just as with housework, sex work, and in-home dependent care, the relative lack of oversight of waxing labor offers some degree of worker autonomy. Small business ownership, for instance, is relatively accessible, with low overhead costs, a number of favorable tax deductions, and the prospect of flexible working hours. The appeal of small business ownership in this realm is clear: in the United States, more than 40 percent of the revenues in hair, nail, and skin services are made by businesses without paid employees, while the average for other industries is 3.5 percent.[55] Self-employment also provides avenues for creative experimentation and expression, as evidenced by aestheticians developing styles such as the Tiffany's Box. So, too, the intimacy and repetition of waxing labor can generate strong bonds between providers and clients.[56]

At the same time, the distinctive closeness of pubic, perineal, and anal waxing can make relations between consumers and service providers complicated, as with other kinds of intimate body care. As sociologist Miliann Kang observes in her path-breaking study of manicuring, body service labor not only entails prolonged physical contact between worker and client but also the management of emotion reflected and generated through that physical contact. Such emotional work is often made more challenging by differences in affluence, language, and/or citizenship status.[57] In the case of total genital depilation, emotional labor is made yet more intense by the pain of the procedure. In one 2002 interview, an aesthetician described a client who

> thrashes around so violently that I'm afraid she's going to break the table and spill hot wax all over both of us. She'll kick her legs, rip the paper table-cover, throw the towels onto the floor, and scream "God-damn you! That hurts!" When it's all over, she gives me a big hug and says "See you in a month."[58]

Indeed, to be "waxed to the max" is sufficiently painful that salons routinely recommend that clients consume alcohol or over-the-counter painkillers prior to treatment: Sherri Shepherd, who received her first Brazilian wax on national television during her popular talk show *The View*, declared the feeling "worse than having a baby." Jonice Padhila, one of the women alternately credited with or blamed for bringing the practice of total genital depilation to the United States, noted that "[s]ometimes I walk by [the waxing room] and hear screams."[59] Due to the intensity of the yanking involved in the procedure, waxing is counter-indicated for individuals using drugs that increase skin sensitivity or easy bruising: Retin-A, Accutane, tetracycline, the blood thinners Coumadin and Warfarin, and some drugs used to treat epilepsy. One salon made light of the pain of the procedure by setting a video montage of clients grunting and cursing during their waxing procedures to the distinctive tune of the "Blue Danube" waltz: rip rip, ouch, ouch.[60]

Again, such complex emotional and physical encounters remain remarkably free of regulatory oversight—including protections for the service providers. No existing state statutes govern acceptable demands on the rate or pace of waxing work itself. One 2004 hair removal manual chirpily noted that a "technician, with training and practice, can become a 'speed waxer,' cutting the typical service time in half and increasing profits."[61] For the self-employed aesthetician or cosmetologist, speed can translate into higher earnings; but for the worker employed by a large franchise or owner-operated salon, expectations of speed can simply be exhausting and debilitating, akin to the strict time-management regimes imposed in other domains of work. Waxers may be subject to repetitive strain injuries and exposure to noxious chemicals as well as thrashing, barking, whimpering clients.[62] It is revealing in this regard that the aestheticians depicted in recent popular representations of Brazilian waxing—from *Sex and the City* to *The Break-Up* to Sherri Shepherd's video diary on *The View*—all appear to be female migrants from Southeast Asia or former Soviet republics.[63] Brazilian waxing, like other kinds of feminized service labor, relies on the mobile women workers moving through the "lower circuits" of global restructuring.[64] It is revealing indeed that when discussing the production of shunned, "wasted," disposable workers in the contemporary global economy, the sociologist Zygmunt Bauman likened these "collateral casualties of progress" to the ritual removal of hair.[65]

Yet popular discussions of waxing focus almost exclusively on the experiences of *clients*, and whether they, consumers, are "enslaved" or "empowered." Although the political status of women and women's bodily self-determination is the recurrent theme of most of these accounts, descriptions of men's genital waxing also have come to emphasize similar themes of domination. When, in late 2007, the writer Christopher Hitchens decided to undergo a

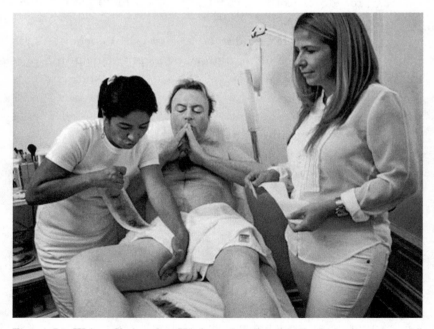

Figure 7.4. Writer Christopher Hitchens describes his "sack, back, and crack" wax in *Vanity Fair*: "The combined effect was like being tortured for information that you do not possess" (December 2007).

Brazilian wax at the hands of New York's J. Sisters, he likened the process to "being tortured for information that you do not possess" (figure 7.4). Hitchens's choice of terms is particularly striking given that the following summer, in the midst of debates over the treatment of U.S. detainees at Guantánamo, he subjected himself to waterboarding in order to determine whether suffocation by water was indeed torturous. (Hitchens ruled that it is.)[66]

Even as recent disputes over the "liberating" or "oppressive" nature of genital waxing tend to erase the broader contexts of the practice, they reproduce twined assumptions about suffering and consent. Whether an act was considered truly "voluntary" affected commentators' perceptions of its violence, and vice versa. What—and who—might get to qualify as suffering would continue to inform evolving practices of hair removal, even as Americans began shifting from sticky waxes to more high-tech solutions.

MAGIC BULLETS

Laser Regulation and Elective Medicine

THE PREVALENCE OF waxing in the early twenty-first century, a method of hair removal with antecedents in the ancient world, highlights a curious fact about Americans' increasingly dogged pursuit of hairless skin: despite decades of experimentation with a staggering array of tools, depilation has remained stubbornly resistant to mechanization. Extracting vast numbers of tiny, embedded objects from the variable surface of the living body continues to present a daunting technical challenge. The arrival of hair removing lasers in the closing years of the twentieth century thus seemed to auger a welcome technological revolution: a way to abolish the time-consuming, skill-intensive, physically taxing labor of manual hair removal. "Instead of painstakingly treating each individual hair," summarized one proponent of laser hair removal in 1991, "a beam of light searches out its target like a 'magic bullet,' treating multiple hairs with a single pulse."[1]

The first such "bullet" approved in the United States for use on humans was a Q-switched neodymium-yttrium-aluminum-garnet (Nd:YAG) laser in 1995, produced by the San Diego-based Thermolase Corporation.[2] The approval followed decades of experimentation: Leon Goldman, a Cincinnati-based physician who died in 1997, is generally credited with first exploring dermatological applications of lasers in the early 1960s.[3] Approved by the Food and Drug Administration in April 1995 on the condition that the words "painless," "permanent," and "long-term" not appear in marketing materials, the technique was a stunning commercial success. Within ten years of its introduction, there were more than 1,566,000 laser hair removal procedures completed in the United States each year: more laser hair removal than liposuctions, rhinoplastic surgeries, eyelid surgeries, and breast augmentations *combined*. Lasers are now used to remove hair from most areas of the body other than the scalp: faces, underarms, backs, pubic regions, legs, chests, abdomens, and arms are all routine targets.[4] By 2006, laser hair removal was the second most prevalent nonsurgical procedure in the country for both men and women (after Botox injections) and *the* most prevalent procedure for customers nineteen to thirty-four years of age.[5]

The technique has been as lucrative as it has been widespread. When Thermolase went public, shares closed the first day at $3.75; within two years share prices leapt to $36.38.[6] A single laser company, the Candela Corporation of Wayland, Massachusetts, reported total revenues of $109.6 million for the nine-month period ending on March 31, 2007. Although such total dollar figures pale when compared to revenues in pharmaceutical products (domestic revenues for Pfizer's cholesterol-lowering drug Lipitor approached $7 billion in the same period), they represented uncommon price-to-earnings ratios for investors. Massachusetts-based Palomar Medical Technologies, for instance, was ranked third on *Business Week*'s 2006 list of one hundred "Hot Growth" companies, after the laser maker's 2005 sales leapt more than 40 percent, to $76.2 million.[7] One industry publication predicted that demand for cosmetic products would continue to grow at a rate of more than 11 percent annually, with nonsurgical products like lasers leading those gains.[8] According to one prominent dermatologist, "nothing on the horizon" threatens lasers' current preeminence in hair reduction: it is "the gold standard, silver and bronze standard right now. There's nothing even close."[9]

The tsunami of laser hair removal at the turn of the twenty-first century arose in part from the same source as the parallel surge in waxing: images of hairlessness promoted in rapidly proliferating media, nestled within a broader expansion of postindustrial service labor. But the growth of laser hair removal also reflects more specific transformations in the legal and economic landscape of American medicine, transformations that generated new unions of science and commerce. Laser consumers readily responded to the promise of scientific solutions to unwanted hair, much as earlier consumers had with glandular extracts and x-ray machines. Yet as before, the emancipation sought through science often turned out to be more complicated than initially hoped.

INNOVATION IN LASER hair removal can be traced to work conducted by subcontractors working for the U.S. Department of Defense. Security specialists sought to develop mobile laser weapons that could operate in deserts and other extreme weather conditions, cooled with air rather than water to enhance their portability and energy efficiency. Tactical laser weapons were troubled both technically and politically, but compact, mobile lasers found successful civilian applications. That success was aided by the profusion of talented physicists in the private sector after the collapse of the Soviet Union, which gutted funding for the physical sciences in Eastern bloc nations. ("Talk about the peace dividend!" one specialist mused when reflecting on Russian physicists' influence on the development of laser hair removal.)[10]

The development and refinement of cutaneous laser applications also was aided by the increasing availability of suitable nonhuman model organisms. Particularly crucial were hairless guinea pigs, bred to contain a mutation first identified in 1978, and a mostly hairless variety of miniature pig, bred from animals imported from Mexico's Yucatan peninsula. Biomedical researchers identified the animals' relatively small size, their "tractability," and their skin's resemblance to human skin as particularly well suited to laboratory conditions. Using guinea pigs and minipigs, investigators were able to test the effects of various laser intensities and pulse widths on living skin.[11]

The diverse hair removing lasers developed through such experiments worked (and still work) in more or less the same way: electromagnetic energy emitted by the laser is absorbed by the melanin in the hair bulb; that energy is converted into heat, which destroys the hair bulb. The whole process relies on calibrated thermal injury, directed by the laser's operator. Lasers of varying wavelengths and frequencies allow practitioners to capitalize on the particular energy absorption tendencies of skin with different levels of melanin. Specialized lasers range from the relatively shallow penetration of the ruby laser (694 nanometer wavelength) to the alexandrite (755 nm), pulsed diode (810 nm), and Nd:YAG laser (1,064 nm), whose wavelengths penetrate the skin to the greatest depth. Flashlamp or Intense Pulsed Light (IPL) devices operate similarly but emit a filtered range of light (515 to 1,200 nm) rather than one specific wavelength (figure 8.1).[12]

The effects of these lasers on tissue, one textbook summarizes, "are analogous to grilling a steak: the first effect is browning of the surface, due to thermal denaturation of hemoglobin and other proteins, followed by sizzling as water is vaporized, followed by shrinkage and charring."[13] The sensations associated with this "charring" can be intense, to put it charitably. Many treatment facilities offer prescriptions of lidocaine to be administered before treatment; some provide intravenous sedation with morphine,

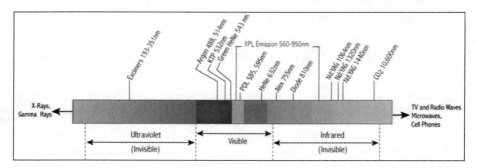

Figure 8.1. The regions of the electromagnetic spectrum used in medical laser applications. (Image from Shino Bay Cosmetic Dermatology, Plastic Surgery, and Laser Institute, Fort Lauderdale, Florida.)

Demerol, and Valium.[14] The goal throughout is to char enough cells to obtain the desired freedom from both hair and the repetitive labor of hair removal while avoiding "excessive injury" to the skin.[15] In early applications of the new technology, avoiding "excessive" injury turned out to be fairly difficult, as the laser could not always distinguish between the melanin in the hair bulb and the melanin in the surrounding skin. The first generation of lasers removed hair most efficiently when the comparative concentration of melanin was much higher in the targeted hair than the surrounding skin tissue: that is to say, on pale skin with dark hair. Flesh with "too much melanin," two physicians wrote in 2002, makes a "poor target for laser energy," since energy is absorbed not only by the melanin in the hair shaft but also by melanin in the adjacent skin.[16]

But precisely how much melanin was "too much"? While relative melanin concentrations were crucial to the safety and efficacy of laser hair removal, some dermatologists recognized the racial prejudices, often unconscious, informing medical norms. To circumvent the clinical inadequacies of the "simple visual assessment of skin color" once used in dermatology, skin physicians promoted adoption of a novel classificatory standard developed by Thomas B. Fitzpatrick of the Harvard Medical School. The Fitzpatrick Skin Phototype scale begins not with physicians' ascriptions (e.g., "too much" or "too little" melanin) but with a questionnaire intended to elicit patients' own self-understandings. Patients respond to experiential criteria such as, "What happens when you stay in the sun too long?" or "What is the color of your skin in areas not exposed to the sun?" On the basis of the patient's answers to such questions, the patient is allotted a score along a spectrum of six photoypes, ranging from Skin Type I ("Very fair skin accompanied by blonde or light red hair . . . never tans, always burns") to Skin Type VI ("Black skin accompanied by black hair and black eyes. Never burns"). "When all else fails," Fitzpatrick liked to tell his residents, "listen to your patient."[17]

Subsequent hair removal devices, referred to by some proponents as "color-blind" lasers, could then be calibrated not by "race"
but by "skin type," using longer wavelengths to try to ameliorate
some of the charring associated with first-generation lasers. (The
longer the wavelength, the more slowly the light energy reaches
into the skin.) The objective, one physician explained, is "to try
to kind of gently cook the whole follicle rather than just cook real
fast."[18] The delay was thought to enable additional external cooling
of the skin, thereby decreasing the risk of thermal injury.[19] Industry
publications happily predicted that the arrival of such customized
laser therapies would lead to special growth in laser hair removal
in "under-developed ethnic markets."[20]

These predictions proved accurate. Clinics designed to cater to
"ethnic markets" began opening around the country in the mid-
2000s. The Feinberg School of Medicine at Northwestern University in Chicago opened a Center for Ethnic Skin; the private
Cultural Cosmetic Medical Spa in Washington, D.C., treated former Miss America Ericka Dunlap, basketball star Alonzo Mourning, and Radio One president Alfred C. Liggins III, among others.
Similar clinics and centers began operating in Philadelphia, New
York, Montclair (New Jersey), and other American cities. Dr. Eliot F. Battle Jr., owner of the Cultural Cosmetic Medical Spa and a
leader in specialized skin care treatment, pointed out that "people
of color represent the fastest growing segment of cosmetic therapy" in the United States.[21]

THE REMARKABLE DIFFUSION of these new tools was made possible by the changing economic and legal context of American
medicine. Beginning early in the 1960s, increased public funding
for poor and elder medical care through Medicare and Medicaid
and a maturing postwar baby boom generation led to growing
concern about a shortage of physicians in the United States. In
response to these concerns, the federal government began pour-
ing money into medical education, which resulted in a doubling
of the annual number of U.S. medical school graduates between

1965 and 1985.[22] The same years witnessed the expansion of the J-1 visa program, founded to enhance medical provision to underserved rural areas. The J-1 program brought rising numbers of international medical students and graduates to the United States for education, residency, and employment.[23] Growth in the medical training and licensing of U.S.-born students, combined with increased migration to the United States by foreign medical graduates, produced a spike in the number of licensed physicians practicing in the United States: there were 148 non–federally employed physicians per 100,000 persons in 1970, but by 2000 there were 288 per 100,000—nearly twice as many.[24]

As it turned out, neither federal nor private expenditures for medical care kept pace with original 1960s projections, leading to a glut of highly trained practitioners. Underemployment produced increased competition among doctors, which in turn generated new strategies to increase demand for medical services. Countries with nationalized health care systems tend to regulate such strategies. In Britain, for example, the state regulates not only the overall intake of new medical specialists but also the number of practitioners working in a given specialty. The United States, however, relies largely on the market to govern such shifts.[25] For some time, the American medical profession maintained an ethic of care explicitly averse to the generation of profit. This professional norm enabled some indirect regulation of medical practice, as physicians who too aggressively sought to expand consumption of their services might be subject to censure from their colleagues. But that professional norm was altered by a series of regulatory shifts in the 1970s. In an effort to rein in galloping health care costs, the Federal Trade Commission began to use existing antitrust law to overturn physicians' self-imposed ban on personal, direct-to-consumer marketing. In *Goldfarb v. Virginia State Bar* (1975), the U.S. Supreme Court held that members of the "learned professions" are subject to the Sherman Antitrust Act, emboldening efforts to overturn professional trade restrictions. Other court decisions similarly collapsed received distinctions between medicine and other trades, forcing professional societies and state licensing boards to loosen their restrictions on individual physicians. This judicial shift hastened physicians' ventures into direct-to-consumer marketing. Newly deregulated physicians, swimming in a hyper-competitive pool of underemployed practitioners, soon began advertising their goods and services in telephone books, on talk show interviews or "infomercials," and through educational seminars.[26]

Increasing competition and decreased regulation resulted in the rise of "medi-spas"—free-standing units that co-opted some elements of the women-run health centers crafted by feminists in the 1970s. An important by-product of that activism was the elevation of women in everyday medical decision making. By the early 1980s, women's concerns were increasingly seen as driving the U.S. health care market; some health care executives deliberately used only female pronouns when referring to their imagined clienteles, in recognition of the fact that "the vast majority of a family's healthcare decisions are made by Mom."[27] Fierce competition for "Moms" with discretionary income led clinics to add features designed to attract women consumers: retail space, beauty services, specialized boutiques, and so on.[28] Once established, such medi-spas organized to defend their position with specialized lobbyists and trade groups. "Now the cat's out of the bag," one physician lamented. "Right now it's anything goes."[29]

Indeed, although laser equipment itself is far more heavily monitored than most other hair removal devices, it is subject to (appallingly) little state, federal, or professional oversight, particularly when used in private offices. Some equipment manufacturers do not allow physicians to purchase their lasers outright, instead requiring leasing arrangements in which physicians pay per-treatment and/or per-month minimums to the manufacturer or dealer. Moreover, some contracts contain "gag" clauses that muffle physicians' ability to discuss negative results with prospective clients, or that bind equipment refunds to a commitment not to publicize reasons for the equipment's return. As a result, reliable comparative data on laser safety and efficacy are difficult to obtain. Even where more stringent reporting and oversight regulations do exist, there is little funding for enforcement. California, which has unusually tough laws concerning laser accreditation and inspection, relegates such practices to the understaffed Enforcement Unit of the state Board of Barbering and Cosmetology. Florida relies on a thinly staffed Board of Medicine with a "backlog of potential disciplinary cases that take an average of nineteen to forty months to resolve."[50] Physicians thus can continue to practice years after formal complaints have been filed challenging their judgment or competence, and machines can remain available for purchase long after consumers experience problems.[51]

The relative laxity of laser regulation also accelerated physicians' investment in procedures perceived as "elective" and "cosmetic." Unlike specialties fettered by single anatomical locations (hearts, noses, etc.), the removal of hair is a flexible area of expertise, with possibilities for expansion across the entire body: one might offer to remove hair from a shin or a chin. While Federal Food and Drug Administration guidelines maintain that lasers must be used by (or used under the direction of) licensed physicians, implementation and enforcement is left to individual states. Application of the FDA mandate therefore varies widely. In California, for example, laser hair removal may be conducted either by a physician or by a registered nurse or physician assistant working in alliance with a physician. In New York, licensed cosmetologists and aestheticians may provide laser hair removal provided that they offer a "clear, distinct disclaimer" that the practice "is not regulated in any way by the Department of State." In Kentucky only licensed physicians may perform the treatment.[52]

In the early 2000s, that regulatory flexibility made laser hair removal a remarkably expedient way for physicians to bring in direct revenue, at least for those who could foot the $69,000 to

$125,000 initial cost of laser equipment.[33] One 2005 review provided a deliberately conservative income projection: "If your laser hair removal service averages four new patients a week, and each patient receives four treatments, that's an average of 16 patients per week after startup. At an average payment of $100 per treatment you'll earn $1,600 per week, or $80,000 annually (assuming that your office is open 50 weeks a year)."[34] So successful were such numbers at enticing nondermatologists into the field of hair removal that the composition of both laser specialties and general practice changed as a result. One laser expert noted that an attendee at a meeting of the American Society for Laser Surgery Medicine in 1991 would have encountered a "smorgasbord" of biologists, general surgeons, gynecologists, and dermatologists; today, in contrast, one would find "90% family physicians."[35] In the trade-show hall of a 2005 meeting of the American Academy of Family Physicians, more than a dozen laser manufacturers staffed booths (figure 8.2).[36]

Physicians caught in these political-economic currents routinely described feeling obligated to provide "spa" services to patients, lest they be dropped out of the increasingly competitive health care market altogether.[37] As one Massachusetts physician grumbled, "I went into medicine to help people and make them feel better, not to do laser hair removal," but "we need to do something to get some cash flow."[38] Other physicians found laser hair removal offered welcome respite from the onerous bureaucracy of health maintenance organizations and capitated insurance plans. "You don't have to deal with the hassle of third-party payers," one physician remarked, when explaining his decision to offer the procedure.[39]

Laser hair removal thus flourished, much like x-ray epilation, by hovering on the edges of professional medicine. While FDA guidelines expressly stipulate that lasers remain under the direction of licensed physicians, specific state regulations vary enormously. (Further confusing the situation, in 2008 the Food and Dug Administration approved the first over-the-counter laser

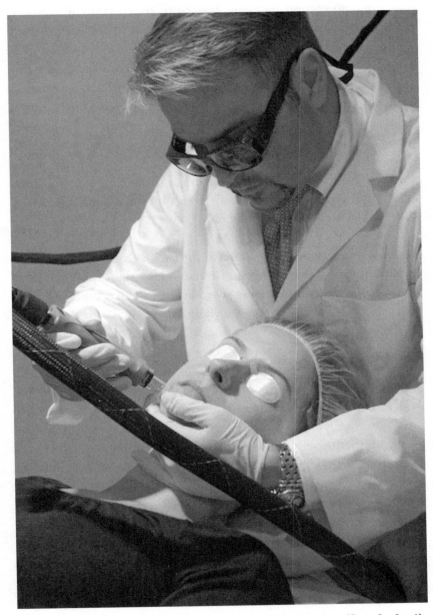

Figure 8.2. A promotional photo of a laser in operation in the office of a family physician in New York; growing numbers of general practitioners began offering laser hair removal in the early 2000s.

hair removal system for home use, the Tria.)[40] Many of the physicians who began offering laser hair removal did so precisely because it was a nonreimbursable "cosmetic" procedure. And physicians' involvement in the work itself was often quite slim: one 2011 study found that most lawsuits based on laser injuries involved a nurse, medical assistant, technician, or other nonphysician operating the laser.[41] As a result, laser hair removal's status as a legitimate medical therapy remained precarious enough to occasion concern among some practitioners. One dermatologist noted that he and others specializing in laser hair removal have been "marginalized": "the real hardcore old school dermatologists would say that we've sold out."[42]

EVEN AS PHYSICIANS were describing themselves as pushed into hair removal by the changing financial realities of medicine, direct-to-consumer advertisements for laser hair removal were tempting Americans to give up their waxes and razors for a more sophisticated, "medical" solution. These advertisements, like earlier promotions for x-ray hair removal, emphasized the laser's emancipating potential: the prospect of ending the repetitive, time-consuming labor of routine hair removal. In most ads, lasers themselves are imperceptible, other than in references to cost (ranging from $75 to $250 per session). Presented instead is the imagined laser client—youthful, thin, smooth-skinned, and sexually desirable. One arresting print advertisement, circulated in *Time Out New York*, the *New York Post*, the *Village Voice*, and other New York media outlets, displayed a pale-skinned, pouty-lipped, sultry-eyed woman gazing directly at the camera. Naked but for a fedora and a strategically placed cat, the ad touts a three-year guarantee on hair removal under the tagline: "We obsess so you won't have to" (figure 8.3).

Other promotions in mainstream media similarly display unclothed or semiclothed women models, posed to accentuate sensual bodily curves and completely hairless white skin, eyes languidly closed or semiclosed. Advertisements featuring men

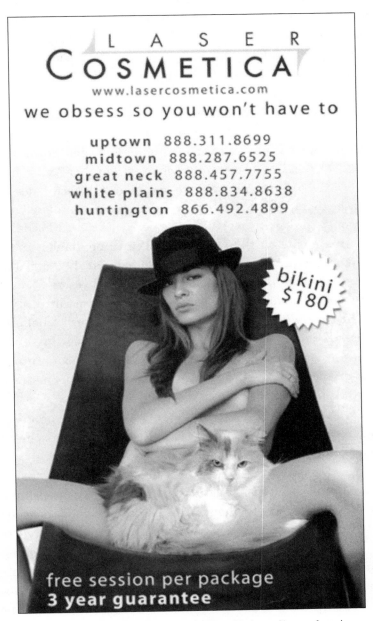

Figure 8.3. A laser promotion run in New York media markets in the 2000s.

usually include a close-up of a lean, chiseled, completely hair-free torso or back, evoking concern about appearing shirtless and "untreated" in public. The "freedom" to be found through laser hair removal predominates online, print, and television advertisements, although freedom *from* what or *to* what is rarely spelled out (figure 8.4).

Consumers evidently found such promotions appealing, as demonstrated by the surge of laser hair removal procedures since 1995 and by the hundreds of testimonials posted online. After "years" of feeling "completely ashamed" by her "very noticeable beard," a thirty-year-old woman from California described her laser therapy as a "life-changing" process, completely worth the money and pain expended.[43] A laser client in Florida, after eight treatments on the face, back, bikini line, hands, and feet, described the process as "EXCRUCIATINGLY painful" ("and I'm no baby about pain"), but praised some of the "awesome" results.[44] A 25-year-old woman in St. Louis described her painful, sixteen-year struggle with body hair and the "tremendous" relief offered by laser therapy, "the best thing I've ever done for myself." After laser treatments, she reported, "I wake up in the morning and touch my face and instead of cringing and feeling disgusted with myself, I smile."[45]

Yet consumers also fell into the gap between promises of "touch-free," lasting hair removal and the realities of sometimes painful, ineffective, and debilitating treatment. One user from New Mexico said that the treatment made her legs feel "like they were on fire." Left with "reddish dark crust[s]," peeling skin, and visible stripes of hypopigmentation, the user reported that she had been "crying and depressed" ever since. Although spared from similar burns, a laser client in Pennsylvania reported feelings of depression. After six seemingly successful laser treatments of her upper lip, the client decided to "try [her] belly line also," to remove the "3 hairs" that bothered her. At the time of her posting to the online forum, she reported "visible hair" growing across her breasts and stomach, as well as new hair growth on her cheeks and

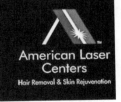

Figure 8.4. "Freedom" through laser hair removal.

chin. Stressing the emotion with capital letters, the user lamented, "I AM DEPRESSED AND SICK OF WHT [SIC] NEVER HAD TO DEAL WITH BEFORE. I WISH I HAD BEEN GREATFUL [SIC]. SORRY GOD."[46]

A distressing *increase* in hairiness after laser therapy, often called "paradoxical laser-induced hair growth stimulation," can also be found in medical literature, along with other adverse effects. Case reports note that the problem is particularly prevalent among "dark-complexioned individuals."[47] A study designed to assess the efficacy of alexandrite laser hair removal for "Asian skin types" concluded by recommending "great caution," for "consistent safety in these darker skin types" has never been demonstrated.[48] A second study found skin changes that included "hypopigmentation, hyperpigmentation, blistering, and scab formation" among dark-skinned patients.[49] A third concluded that rates of complication increase "as skin pigment increases."[50] Such effects are particularly "disconcerting," the two authors summarized, "because of the difficulty in identifying the exact etiology."[51]

Similar complications were reported by two practitioners treating a "27-year-old Indian woman" who had received laser hair removal on her face: "One day after treatment she presented with areas of hyperpigmentation with a thin membrane of superficially desquamating skin over small portion [sic] of her face." (The injuries do not appear to have dulled her desire for laser therapy.)[52] These findings echoed accounts in popular media, such as that of 31-year-old Josabet Tecat-Suarez, a New Jersey resident who purchased laser hair removal, performed by her gynecologist, in preparation for her 2002 wedding. In the middle of her treatment, Tecat-Suarez's skin started to sizzle. Afterward, Tecat-Suarez described her skin as resembling a "tick-tack-toe board," with oozing wounds dotting her brown complexion. She then underwent a year of chemical peels—at $220 each—in order to undo the damage.[53] Transgender activist Andrea James, founder of a well-trafficked website devoted to hair removal, publicized the dangers of lasers to "dark skin" in a graphic 2008 video.[54] Disgruntled and maimed clients continue to post complaints on consumer and beauty websites, where they often connect with lawyers willing to represent them in personal injury claims (figure 8.5).

DESPITE THE EVIDENT risks of lasting injury presented by cutaneous laser therapy, and the particular risks posed to people of color, laser hair removal remains the "gold standard" of hair removal in the twenty-first century, an emblem of emancipation through medical progress. Strikingly, recent popular debate over lasers tends to focus not on their safety or efficacy but on the boundaries of their "medically necessary" application. The efforts of two transwomen incarcerated in men's prisons in Massachusetts to gain access to laser hair removal, as treatment for their diagnosed gender dysphoria, triggered ugly public debate. Their legal right to medical treatment was not in doubt: the Supreme Court's affir-

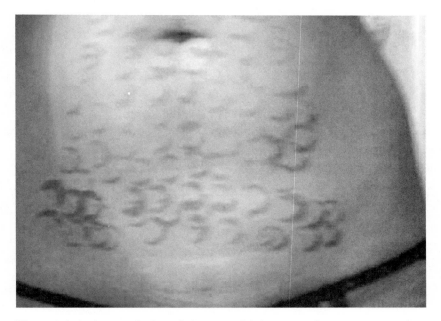

Figure 8.5. An image of a laser hair removal injury, posted to a consumer advocacy website in 2010.

mation of prisoners' rights to "adequate medical care" was established in 1976 and extended in 1993; denial of such care has been found to violate the Eighth Amendment's prohibition on "cruel and unusual punishment."[55] Rather, at stake in the Massachusetts cases was for whom unwanted hair constituted real suffering, and, by extension, whether and for whom the application of lasers constituted legitimate medical need. Concern about the "expense to taxpayers" of treatment merely exposed the underlying valuations of particular bodies.[56]

Thus, even as laser hair removal proliferated among American consumers—evolving into a personal "lifestyle decision" that required medical supervision—conflict persisted over the meanings of the medically "serious."[57] Hair removal remained a site of legal, professional, and popular contestation of those meanings: whether relief from hair merited deliberate "charring" of tissue. The next logical step in this vision of enhancement would be to try to eliminate the need for hair removal altogether.

[9]

"THE NEXT FRONTIER"

Genetic Enhancement and the End of Hair

IN 1990, THE U.S. Department of Energy, the National Institutes of Health, and a company called Celera Genomics began a formal collaboration to determine the sequences of the three billion chemical base pairs comprising human DNA and to identify its roughly twenty-five thousand genes, or functional segments. Committed from the outset to transferring the knowledge and tools it developed to private sector companies, the collaboration, officially known as the Human Genome Project, kindled the rapid growth of commercial biotechnology in the United States: according to some reports, related revenues from publicly traded U.S. companies rose from just over $8 billion in 1992 to more than $28 billion in 2001. Although the project was estimated to last fifteen years, international cooperation sped completion. A working draft of the genome was announced in 2001, and the project was completed in 2003.[1]

The effort triggered vigorous discussion of the ethics and politics of human genetic research, and the potential consequences of future genetic enhancement. Politicians, theologians, regulators, journalists, and academics all joined the debates.[2] Some social scientists proposed that the rise of genomics indicated a qualitative shift in understandings of human (and nonhuman) variation: a movement from imagining difference at the "molar" level of limbs, organs, and hormones to the "molecular" level of proteins,

171

genes, and genomes. Various conferences and publications wrestled with the implications of the "molecularization" or "geneticization" of society.[3]

Meanwhile, investigations into some "genetically guided" products sprang up largely free from scrutiny and debate. In an inchoate field variously referred to as "cosmeceuticals," "vanity genetics," or "Dermagenetics," researchers began applying techniques gleaned from human genetics to the improvement of "beauty and wellness."[4] Already, consumers with the means to do so might purchase skin care formulations that link specific combinations of active ingredients to the results of personal genetic tests. More intriguing still are efforts to actually alter cellular machinery, based on the discovery that double-stranded molecules of ribonucleic acid (RNA) can selectively silence the expression of targeted genes. Experimental tools of RNA-interference (RNAi) in various stages of development address everything from hair luster to iris color. For example, in 2003 the publicly traded cosmetics company Avon, Inc., filed for patent protection on gene silencing techniques for the reduction of "unwanted pigmentation." Picking up on the technique's potential, several small start-ups and larger biotechnology firms sought ways to use gene silencing to retard or arrest the growth of unwanted hair. So promising did such products appear at one point that in 2004 the global pharmaceutical company Merck paid $1.1 billion to acquire a leader in RNAi development, Sirna Therapeutics: more than twice Sirna's stock value at the time.[5]

If realized, efforts to alter hair growth at the genetic level portend a quiet but profound shift in practices of hair removal, and in the history of body modification more broadly. For such strategic genetic interference holds the prospect of erasing some phenotypic characteristics altogether, as in the aforementioned effort to alleviate "unwanted pigmentation." While it is too early to know whether or when such products might be brought to market, RNAi-based hair removal would spell a marked departure from lasers, depilatories, waxes, and razors, in deliberately re-configuring the architecture of living cells. (X-rays also mutated genes, but those changes were an unintended consequence of their use in hair removal.) Moreover, given the prevalence of hair removal in contemporary America, RNAi solutions to unwanted hair could bring genetic engineering into Americans' daily lives in an unprecedented way.[6] Indeed, the domestic market for gene-based hair retardation is larger even than the sizable market for new techniques of hair *growth*: not only do more Americans seek to remove than add hair, but American consumers also tend to want to grow hair only on the top of the head, whereas hair might be removed from almost everywhere else on the body.[7] Further-more, because siRNA hair retardation is not affected by pigmen-tation levels, there should be no demonstrable difference in safety or efficacy from one skin tone to the next—an obvious advantage over the current "gold standard," laser hair reduction.[8] For these reasons, gene-based hair removal has the potential to "domesti-cate" complex bioengineering, much as the introduction of elec-tric lighting paved the way for reliance on other electrical devices within the household.[9]

The fact that commercialization has not yet been achieved, however, suggests the weight of divisions between cosmetic or lifestyle indications and "real" medical necessity, divisions that direct pharmaceutical research. Even as third-party payers, gov-ernment regulators, consumer watch-dog groups, and journal-ists heap blame on physicians and pharmaceutical companies for steering American medicine toward frivolous "lifestyle" thera-pies, evidence gathered from researchers themselves indicates a striking hesitancy to engage in the low-prestige work of hair re-moval. As a result, consumers seeking new therapies for their un-wanted hair are left languishing.

RIBONUCLEIC ACID INTERFERENCE burst onto the international scientific scene in the late 1990s and has remained on the fore-front of research since. RNAi is based on short, double-stranded molecules (dsRNA) whose sequence of nucleotides (adenine, cytosine, guanine, uracil) matches the targeted gene. Once inside a cell, the dsRNA molecule is cleaved into shorter segments, roughly twenty-one nucleotides long, called "short interfering RNAs" (siRNAs). These siRNAs then activate complexes within the cell to bind to matching sequences of single-stranded messenger RNA (mRNA), typically cleaving the mRNA and attenuating expression of the gene from which the mRNA came. In this way, RNAi can be used to silence a particular gene, without apparent effect on other genes (figure 9.1).[10]

The potential applications of the tool are countless. By hindering or "knocking down" a specific gene and observing how the cell responds, researchers can now quickly validate gene function and examine the therapeutic value of suppressing a particular gene. In theory, any gene whose expression is linked to a specific disease—diabetes, breast cancer, Alzheimer's—could be targeted and silenced. Such potent possibilities attracted zealous commentary. In 2002, *Science* magazine dubbed RNAi the event of the year. In 2003, *Fortune* magazine christened RNAi the life sciences' next "billion dollar breakthrough," while *Wired* magazine termed it "the biggest boon biotech has seen in decades." In 2004 *Nature* magazine devoted an entire issue to the subject.[11] This enthusiastic media reception was matched by more rare recognition: in 2006, the Nobel Prize in Physiology or Medicine was awarded to Andrew Z. Fire and Craig C. Mello for their contribu-

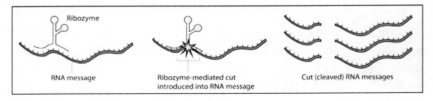

Figure 9.1. "A ribozyme binds to a specific mRNA, cleaves it, and thus prevents it from functioning." (From "RNAi Therapeutics: How Likely, How Soon?" *PLoS Biology* [2004].)

tion to the development of RNAi, a mere eight years after their first publication on the topic.[12]

In the midst of feverish interest in RNAi came the publication of several major studies correlating human hair growth and color with identifiable genetic variants.[13] When subsequent findings suggested the efficacy of siRNAs in regulating the expression of specific hair-related genes, financial and intellectual resources began flowing toward the molecular biology of hair.[14] Researchers and investors recognized that inhibiting the genes responsible for hair growth and follicle integrity could result in a permanent, painless—and wildly lucrative—form of hair removal. By 2006, several different avenues of siRNA-mediated hair retardation were being pursued.

Years passed, however, and RNAi-based hair removers remained stalled in the development stage (at the time of this book's publication, no such "gene creams" had yet reached the market). Through interviews with company executives, investors, industrial and academic molecular biologists, biochemists, and investigative dermatologists in the field, I tried to learn what the next frontier of hair removal techniques might be—at least as far as the proprietary and competitive nature of drug development would allow.[15]

Several interviewees pointed out substantial technical challenges to successful drug delivery: getting the hair-retarding molecule through the skin, down the hair shaft, into the cell, and reliably to the desired target.[16] Yet nearly all of the industry leaders interviewed insisted that such technical challenges were relatively minor. Of far greater hindrance to successful commercialization of these tools, they proposed, was a form of self-policing ongoing in the pharmaceutical industry, which limited attention to new hair removing therapies. Understanding this self-monitoring requires consideration of the distinctive regulatory climate of drug development in the contemporary United States.

THE U.S. FOOD and Drug Administration's efforts are governed by the 1938 Food, Drug, and Cosmetic Act—an act forged in no small part in response to injuries and deaths associated with the toxic thallium acetate depilatory, Koremlu. The act, as we have seen, defines "cosmetics" as articles "applied to the human body" for "cleansing, beautifying, promoting attractiveness, or altering the appearance." Under the act, reporting on cosmetics is almost entirely voluntary. Objects classified as "drugs," on the other hand, those "intended to affect the structure or function of the body," are subject to carefully managed federal reviews of safety, efficacy, and manufacturing processes.[17] Explicitly designed to affect underlying structure, RNAi-based hair removers would therefore be subject to levels of FDA oversight that razors, depilatories, and waxes all avoid.

Just as the FDA distinguishes between cosmetics and drugs, it also maintains distinct approval processes for drugs for "serious" and "nonserious" conditions. Drugs designed for what are widely seen as "elective" uses, such as the alleviation of acne, are referred to as "aesthetic" or "lifestyle" indications. They are subject to stricter testing and approval regimes than drugs intended for, say, the progressive neurodegenerative condition known as amyotrophic lateral sclerosis, or "Lou Gehrig's disease." These regulatory distinctions—between drug and cosmetic and between serious and elective—shape the course of drug development. As one RNAi researcher put it, "if you are going after a lifestyle drug, a non-disease indication, you have to be so incredibly safe that you're not ever going to have a problem." "FDA people," he continued, always calculate in terms of "risk and benefit": "if you're not really improving someone's health and there's any risk at all, [they're] not going to approve it."[18] A researcher at a large multinational biotech company concurred: "it depends on the type of drug how safe it has to be. . . . [I]f you want more or less hair growth, you don't want your adrenal glands dying, you don't want your white blood cell count to plummet. So you have to have a very, very squeaky-clean safety bar."[19] The perceived severity of the patient's (or consumer's) suffering, in other words, determines the important regulatory distinction between "elective" and "lifesaving" therapies. "Lifestyle" drugs—those deemed optional—face higher regulatory hurdles and a slower route to market.

The curious feature of regulatory relations among suffering, seriousness, and "elective" treatments is that these determinations are interconnected, established in hierarchical relation to one another. The seriousness of a given drug's adverse effects is weighed not against some fixed standard (such as whether a dosage of one tablespoon kills eight or nine out of ten laboratory mice in controlled studies), but, as the remarks about "risk and benefit" above suggest, against beliefs about the severity of the initial condition being treated. Intravenous chemotherapy drugs, for instance, carry potent adverse effects, but through the drug approval process those effects have been judged preferable to existing cancers. Similarly, the severity of the initial disease or condition is established comparatively, vis-à-vis the agency's assessment of just what level of "adverse effects" it is willing to tolerate in the effort to ameliorate it. "Seriousness," in other words, is a relational attribute rather than an inherent property.[20]

Leaders in the development of RNAi hair therapies were quick to emphasize the relational character of the FDA's understandings of the serious and the trivial. One interviewee exemplified the point by describing Allergan, Inc.'s application for the use of botulinum toxin as a muscle relaxant for children with cerebral palsy. According to the interviewee, an FDA advisory panel dismissed that application as a "lifestyle issue" (and hence under the threshold for drug risk in children), although the agency approved the same medication's use in reducing fine facial lines in adults, and the same company's new remedy for "inadequate" eyelashes, Latisse. The interviewee concluded from this example that the line between lifestyle indication and serious medical need was flexible, shaped by "general cultural shift[s]."[21]

The contingency of the medically "serious" was emphasized by others. One molecular biologist proposed that distinctions between "lifestyle" concerns and "more serious disease" are governed by "perception," perceptions that drug companies deliberately manipulate.[22] He continued, "[T]his is made very clear by Viagra [Pfizer's blockbuster erectile dysfunction drug]. . . .

[S]omehow, they were able to spin going after people's sex lives as being a serious medical indication. And I think that that's changing the landscape."[23] "There are," he noted, "big time lobbyists that work on this stuff."[24] In his company's case, consultants recommended "go[ing] through something like hirsutism first . . . a medical indication," and only then moving "into a broader market."[25] The former CEO of a small start-up and current biotech investor agreed. The goal is "to make it a medical and ethical imperative—creating categories, creating needs. The whole ball of wax is about shaping what necessity is." "Generally speaking," he concluded, "it takes about three years to shape a category."[26]

That the clinicians, molecular biologists, investors, and company executives in the midst of drug development see the designation "serious medical indication" as mutable is not shocking. Described here is a phenomenon so common that critics have given it a name of its own: "medicalization," the repositioning of social concerns as medical conditions, to the benefit of drug and device manufacturers and collaborating physicians.[27] Although often lambasted as an effect of post–World War II consumer capitalism, medicalization is not a new phenomenon, as the examples of hypertrichosis and hirsutism make plain. What has changed in recent years is not the sudden entry of profit into medicine, or a radical shift among physicians from attending to "real" disease to treating fictive "lifestyle" concerns, but the scale and speed at which processes of medicalization (or "biomedicalization") now unfold. Phalanxes of specialized consultants, market analysts, brand specialists, academic researchers, celebrity spokespeople, patient advocacy groups, and bloggers all now participate in moving the legitimizing mantle of medical "seriousness" from one location to another.[28]

The more unexpected point here is that drug developers, too, experience themselves as suffering on the margins of this process. Indeed, all twenty-five people interviewed for this chapter spoke to the perceived seriousness (or lack thereof) of unwanted hair as influencing their work. Despite clear market incentives for developing effective depilatory products—after all, most Americans past the age of puberty routinely use one or more—scientists, clinicians, and executives continually insisted that pharmaceutical companies were *reluctant* to pursue new hair removal therapies. Even as critics inveigh against physicians and pharmaceutical companies for pushing vanity over cures for "more serious" diseases, these RNAi researchers and company executives instead highlighted consequential forms of self-monitoring within the pharmaceutical industry—a collective distaste for research into medications having to do with body hair.

INTERVIEWEES PROPOSED THAT hesitancy about work on drugs for body hair stems from pharmaceutical corporations' concerns about public image: as one scientist said, "[T]he mission statements [of drug companies] are all about improving the lives of people. Improving health care, you know, and making disease ameliorated. . . . [T]here's sort of a stigma if you're a pharmaceutical company and you're not looking at life-threatening disease or life-altering disease."[29] "[I]f you are just trying to remove people's hair," another reported, "that's considered very aesthetic" and "not very worthwhile."[30] According to several interview participants, large pharmaceutical companies diverged from large cosmetics manufacturers in this respect, since the latter did not have to worry about the gravitas of their corporate missions. One RNAi researcher reported being repeatedly approached by cosmetic industry representatives.

> And I tell them, you know, look we're just not very interested. But I say if you were willing to pay us obscene amounts of money to help you and then we could use that money, we might be interested. And the funny thing is that that doesn't turn them off at all. . . . [They say] "what you have, it doesn't have to work very well. It only has to work a tiny bit."[31]

Multinational cosmetic companies were said to be more willing than drug companies to pursue therapies lacking efficacy.

A general unwillingness to be associated with treatments for non-life-threatening illness was further said to tar the whole field of dermatology, which one investor bluntly described as "not sexy."[32] Few large pharmaceutical companies maintain research units dedicated to new dermatological products, despite wide markets for new products and a relative lack of competition. "Dermatologic indications are unique" within the pharmaceutical industry, another interviewee noted:

> You gotta be a lifestyle company. And Allergan [maker of Botox] is the only one that kind of goes there. Nobody else really goes in for lifestyle drugs. They might if it's an alternative indication, but they're not going to have a big group working on a lifestyle drug.[33]

Such reluctance to pursue "derm" drugs puzzled some interviewees. As one company executive reflected, "[Y]ou know, when you think of the skin as the largest organ in the body on math alone all drugs should be [dermatologic] drugs."[34] As another investigative dermatologist jokingly put it, when comparing the level of research on skin medications to the level conducted on male impotence: "[M]y organ is bigger than your organ."[35] One "derm" company executive directed the conversation to a recent medical study, which found that patients with visible skin conditions reported a greater detrimental impact on quality of life than patients with hypertension, angina, or asthma. The executive shook her head while recounting the findings, noting that most pharmaceutical investors and executives just don't take skin seriously enough.[36]

Of course, professionals' claims of marginality must always be considered with several grains of salt—particularly given the financial value of "underdog" branding.[37] Examples of substantial intellectual and financial investment in aesthetic dermatology abound. In 2006, the Johns Hopkins University Medical School formed an alliance with a New York company called Klinger Advance Aesthetics, a subsidiary of luxury goods conglomerate LVMH. In exchange for underwriting, medical school faculty members evaluate products and help the company develop "best practices" for its chain of medi-spas. Similarly, the Weill Cornell Medical College's Department of Dermatology established a "skin wellness center," funded with $7 million from cosmetics giant Clinique Laboratories, Inc., whose name and products were to be displayed prominently. Meanwhile, individual dermatologists routinely act as paid spokespeople for cosmetic products at scientific and professional meetings, often without disclosure of their financial ties to companies.[38] Investors, too, do not appear to be shy about pursuing opportunities in the aesthetic market: at a 2009 investment conference sponsored by Goldman Sachs, events on aesthetic medicine were standing room only.[39] One former executive insisted that investors ultimately follow "business plans and market analyses," not inchoate concerns about the respectability of a company's mission and purposes.[40]

For all the undeniable influence of quantitative market analyses, however, the more intangible role of stigma remained consequential here. Some respondents proposed that the study of hair removal was aversive to drug developers because it meant risking their own professional marginalization—a concern in fields of science and business that depend on the successful maintenance of social networks and reputation.[41] Others expressed reservations based on their personal calculations of ethical value. "To me," explained one Boston-based researcher, "a normal growing hair is not a disease. I'm a doctor and a scientist and I'm like, well, why should I do that?" According to the researcher, a woman colleague eventually helped persuade him that the work was, as he put it, truly "worth doing."[42] Questions of worth, often framed explicitly in terms of cost and benefit, informed numerous comments. At the end of the day, one leading skin biologist noted,

referring to the widespread use of animal models in dermatological studies, "it's sort of hard to justify killing dogs and animals for
hair research."

> You can see if you're doing . . . multiple sclerosis re-
> search and lupus research and cancer research and
> you feel like, okay, that's a good cost/benefit if you
> have to do that. But for skin research, killing hun-
> dreds of animals, it's just hard to justify it from an
> ethical—at least in my own mind—an ethical stand-
> point. . . . [P]eople like to feel that what they're doing
> is—the cost/benefit is worth it, that the chance of—
> that this really will help humanity to the point where
> it's worth sacrificing an animal for.[43]

Others expressed similar squeamishness about work on body hair,
to the point of stumbling when trying to articulate their reasons
for pursuing the topic. "I'm just so fascinated by the follicle, you
know," said one investigator:

> I'm not—certainly not driven by wanting to cure
> bald—you know, people don't—I mean, you know,
> I don't—so people don't realize about science that
> you don't really usually have that kind of a goal, you
> know, that you're kind of—you're going to get there,
> but it's not because you're trying to focus so hard
> around one thing. I know it's hard to explain.[44]

Even pharmaceutical companies have learned to narrate
their research in deliberate ways. When asked why biotechnology venture capitalists might have qualms about funding hair-
related RNAi research, given the apparent blockbuster potential
of such drugs, one molecular biologist replied that it's "the aes-
thetic-ness of it. . . . [A]ll of the other diseases we were working on were life threatening, so it's hard to make that fit into

the ethos of a company, when you have a division that is not doing that."[45] His start-up handled that dilemma by discussing the other diseases, such as melanoma, that might be addressed once they figured out how to deliver short interfering RNAs to the hair follicle. Similarly, when established pharmaceutical companies with known hair removing agents in their portfolios abandon work on hair removal, they are careful to explain their decision making in ways that foreground the distinction between serious and trivial commitments. When Quest PharmTech, Inc., concluded work on one of its candidates for hair removal, they reported that the decision was made "in order to accelerate Quest's focus on oncology."[46] When Merck closed its dermatology division after acquiring Sirna's hair targets for more than $1 billion, one online commentator concluded that they decided to "pursu[e] the oncology track" for "obvious reasons": "I don't think researching how to get rid of unwanted hair was on their priority list."[47]

FACING COMPANIES AND researchers who often belittle their concerns with hair, consumers eager—if not desperate—for new therapies sometimes depict corporate capitalism itself as the obstacle to treatment. In one of the liveliest of multiple English-language websites dedicated to sharing information about unwanted hair and its removal, contributors closely followed developments in siRNA-mediated hair retardation. Some speculated that large cosmetic and personal care product manufacturers deliberately stymie pharmaceutical research in the area, in order to maintain a corner on existing hair removal technologies. One contributor, Eddy, proposed that if a company actually developed "a 'magic bullet' product" like RNAi drugs, the "big boys like Gillette" might fear the threat to their market in razors, blades, and shaving creams: "what woman in her right mind wouldn't use it on her legs, underarms, etc. to avoid the sometimes daily chore of shaving?" The shaving conglomerate would therefore have two options, in Eddy's view:

1. Partner up with Sirna/Quest to assist in funding/developing/marketing the new product in return for royalties on sales. Still profits from their razor/shaving cream divisions will go down as less are demanded, factories close, and P&G employees lose jobs. . . .

OR

2. Us[e] the billions of dollars at their disposal to buy the patent/rights to sell the product from Sirna/Quest, and bury the product preventing its release . . . keeping their stranglehold on the shaving/razor market where it is (very healthy at the moment, have you seen the cost of Mach 3 blades!?!). . . . and forcing the public to continue their lifelong addiction to razors/shaving creams.

Eddy concluded that "keeping a stranglehold" on new research seemed the more likely path.[48] Another contributor echoed Eddy's suspicion of corporate motives.

I loathe conspiracy theories in general, but not in this case. Well, it's not even a conspiracy theory, actually. It's just plain and simple capitalism. Companies are not here to help people, they're here to make money. I'm pretty sure that companies like Gilette [sic] are willing to pay a lot for a patent for a product that could virtually wipe them off the market.[49]

In sharp contrast to those feminist social scientists who attribute intensifying norms of hairlessness to capitalism's need to push new products, according to these consumer advocates, corporate avarice *inhibits* rather than drives innovation in the realm of hair removal.

FOR ALL THE conspiratorial tone of many of the discussions, these web commentators were correct about the core point: technical solutions to unwanted hair have advanced no further than lasers, which remain expensive, painful, and potentially injurious. None of the numerous alternatives proposed has established proof of efficacy: microwave therapies, electrified dermal patches, dietary supplements like spearmint tea, saw palmetto, soy milk, or turmeric powder. For all the hype about the "molecularization" or "geneticization" of society, unwanted hair is still treated with twined thread, sticky wax, and hand-held tweezers, not with RNA interference. Hair's status as a serious or trivial concern, its relative worthiness or unworthiness as an object of study, continues to shape the tools brought to bear on its removal.

Meanwhile, as one siRNA researcher noted, more and more people—around the globe, he stressed—approach body hair "as something they want to control, rather than something they kind of have to put up with": "I think hair is the next frontier where it's this kind of natural thing that people say, well, why do I have to put up with it on my body?"[50] Management of the living body remains the frontier of freedom.

CONCLUSION:
WE ARE ALL PLUCKED

AMERICANS ARE NOT born averse to body hair. Nor is any particular group responsible for all the plucking, waxing, shaving, and lasering evident today. Rather than demonstrating the innate appeal of fur-free skin or a conspiracy designed to infantilize women, the rise of hair removal over the last century could be said to reflect broader sea changes in American social and economic life: the convergence of shifting gender roles, immigration patterns, labor practices, manufacturing processes, domestic arrangements, media flows, racial prejudices, military endeavors, scientific discoveries, and commercial innovations. Over time, hairlessness, once perceived as a characteristic "deficiency" of the continent's indigenous peoples, became normalized—a persistent standard of health, beauty, cleanliness, and desirability.

When asked, however, Americans tend to downplay the influence of such norms and values. Instead, they attribute their own hair removal practices to "personal" goals of increased attractiveness, elevated self-esteem, and enhanced sexual pleasure. We might see in that fact another historical development: the increasing significance of concepts of personal choice in American political life. Nourished by pervasive commercial media, the opacity of global commodity chains, and consistently lax regulation of so-called elective care, ever more emphasis is placed on individual "freedom." And, whether one engages in hair removal or deliberately rejects reigning norms, management of the hairy body has become one more way to exercise that freedom. Shave or wax, laser or pluck: we are empowered to decide, and responsible for our own outcomes.

Students of recent political theory might recognize this trajectory as part of a larger phenomenon: a "liberalization" of the institutions, procedures, and tactics of governance. As political theorists have argued, where once populations were managed through the application of external force (public beheadings, floggings, deprivations of food or water), control in more liberal contexts is distributed and internalized: *self*-management is the name of the game. Indeed, as obligations for health, education, employment, and other elements of social welfare continue to shift from states to markets, a process often called "neoliberalism," the governed are increasingly called to monitor and "maximize" their lives.[1]

Of course, recent U.S. history offers numerous glaring exceptions to this trajectory—conditions in which rule is not devolved to individuals but instead concentrated, hierarchal, and "stuck." Following philosopher Michel Foucault, we might call these conditions, such as the forcible detention ongoing at Guantánamo Bay or the marked expansion of maximum-security incarceration since the 1970s, "states of domination."[2] But in this age of personal responsibility, even states of domination often reveal concern with the psychic and emotional dimensions of rule, with the *inner* management of conduct. One of the distinguishing characteristics of the forced shaving conducted at Guantánamo, for example, is that, like waterboarding, it leaves no visible marks on the body. Such "stealth" techniques, political scientist Darius Rejali has argued, are a hallmark of torture in contemporary democracies. Internal discipline—invisible intervention—is paramount, in states of domination as in practices of freedom.[3]

Put another way, individual choice has become the very vehicle of political control. The more invested we become in "optimizing" individual health and well-being, the more thoroughly do we embody the ebbs and flows of rule. Seen in this light, the waxing, shaving, lasering, and plucking discussed in previous chapters all appear not merely as curious cultural developments but as paradigmatic "practices of the self": the ongoing efforts of personal transformation that, according to Foucault, actually serve as the capillaries of modern power.

GIVEN THE INEXTRICABILITY of personal choice and techniques of power, concluding this study by staking out a position "for" or "against" hair removal would make little sense. As several other accounts of contemporary body modification emphasize, denouncing specific techniques as "oppressive" (or praising them as liberating) misses the key point: these techniques are themselves producing us as individuals tasked with such incessant evaluations.[4] But if not a clear position "for" or "against" particular practices of hair removal, what else might be gleaned from this history? Let me offer three observations—what might be called the "take-home points."

First, I hope that this study deepens consideration of the "upstream" production and "downstream" effects of other forms of body modification. To date, scholarly and popular discussions of technologies of enhancement have tended to concentrate on the site of consumption, on the ramifications of adoption or refusal for individual users. How anabolic steroids might affect the Olympic athlete, how prescription stimulants might affect the college student, how "vaginal rejuvenation" surgery might affect the middle-aged woman: these are the recurrent tropes of ethical concern.

To be sure, a fair number of critics have underscored the potential for increased social stratification presented by the diffusion of enhancement technologies—namely, the prospect of increased discrimination against "unenhanced" humans.[5] The point here is related, but distinct: that the stratifications produced by enhancement are not limited to matters of access. Inequities are propagated well before and well after instances of distribution and use. From the scores of sheep and pigs slaughtered to produce a single dram of gland extract to the thousands of electronics factory workers recruited to assemble home laser devices, from waterways filled with the effluvia of chemical depilatories to air polluted with the belching smoke of petroleum refineries, this book shows how evolving habits of self-management among the privileged rely on and foment new ways of consuming and discarding the lives of others. The uneven effects of "personal" enhancement are distributed broadly, temporally and geographically.[6] Those uneven effects, moreover, are routinely excluded from ethical and political debate.[7] *Plucked* is, first and foremost, a call to remember those excluded others: the staggering volumes of sweat and blood and imagination and fear expended to produce a single hairless chin.

But this is not a call to simply transfer attention from the smooth surfaces of advanced technologies to their hairy, sticky underpinnings. Nor is the goal to shift the analytical gaze from spectacular, relatively rare procedures (face transplants! brain implants!) to more routine, "boring" kinds of bodily management.[8] Rather, the point, the second observation of this book, is that surfaces and underpinnings, the spectacular and the boring, are inextricably intertwined. The boundaries of "serious" bioethical concerns, and of medical "necessity," are continuously remade, symbolically and materially, in relation to the trivial and the superfluous. Much as masculinity co-constitutes femininity or the human co-constitutes the animal, the serious and the trivial are predicated on one another, even while continuously excluded from one another. And, as we have seen, the mutual constitution of essential therapy and elective enhancement requires labor—labor concretized in things like homemade depilatories and prescription hormones, trichometers and hirsutism charts, board certifications and animal use protocols.

The stakes of that labor are obviously high: some experiences of suffering become meaningful, and others are expelled from moral and political concern. When Jefferson and other naturalists scrutinized Indians' repeated "mutilations" of their beards, when Havelock Ellis and other sexologists correlated "excessive" facial hair with criminal behavior, when Betty Friedan and others scolded unshaven activists for veering from the "proper" concerns of second-wave feminism, they were asserting at once the meanings of real suffering and the limits of political inclusion. Such assertions gain much of their potency, this study further suggests, from their tacitness, from the seeming self-evidence of lines between the vital and the trivial. As the use of forced shaving at Guantánamo makes brutally clear, the fact that hair removal is usually conducted without much fanfare, far from the klieg lights of scholarly and popular attention, is precisely what makes it so politically (or "biopolitically") potent.[9] If the work of Foucault teaches us anything, it is that power is working most effectively (and critical scrutiny might be fruitfully concentrated) where activities seem most innocuous.

It may be tempting to hope that better science, improved technology, or more enlightened law eventually will resolve skirmishes over the definition of suffering. Whether forced shaving truly is torturous, whether gender dysphoria merits surgical intervention, whether laboratory animals experience emotional pain: the yearning for expert resolution of such conflicts is understandable. Indeed, the rise of new professions and sub-professions claiming authority over legitimate complaint is a hallmark of our political condition.[10] But determinations of real suffering will never be fixed, once and for all. We are mistaken if we imagine that enhanced technical knowledge or more skillful regulation might set bright, clear lines between the superfluous and the truly necessary. Such lines are merely "alibis," Donna Haraway reminds us, in that they act to conceal our complicity in separating lives that matter from lives that do not.[11] That complicity, the pervasiveness of power, is the third major observation of the book: we are compelled to live within its flows, each in our own mortal way. Even if we never tweeze another hair from another body, we are plucked.

But that take-home point need not be depressing. For the history of hair removal points to the broad, unsettling consequences of the seemingly insignificant act of separating self from other. That work is never complete: the very boundaries of our bodies, to say nothing of the limits of empathy and political action, are, and may be, continually remade.[12] Perhaps it is this openness, this fragility, that has for so long animated hair, that made it a matter of concern to presidents and protestors, scientists and theologians, artists and pornographers: the fundamental unruliness of life.

Acknowledgments

OVER THE MANY years that it took to complete this book, I delivered quite a few public lectures on hair removal. Each time I did, someone, often more than one person, would ask me to explain what led me to the topic. So, too, whenever I sent out manuscripts for formal scholarly review, one or more referees would inquire about my "personal connection" to hair removal. A reviewer for this press similarly encouraged me to say a few words about how I "came to the subject" of body hair.

The inquisitiveness itself is noteworthy. This book is the third work of nonfiction I've published. I've also churned out a fair number of articles, reviews, and professional talks on other themes. With a single exception (a friendly request, during my doctoral defense, to describe the autobiographical relevance of my dissertation topic), on no other subject has anyone inquired about my "personal" investment in the research at hand. With body hair, though, interest in my back story has been inescapable.

What is it that people want to know, exactly? I've never been able to discern. Are they wondering about my political biases? About my disciplinary training or expertise? About whether I shave my legs? The confusion is compounded by the ambiguity of any project's origins. Where and how was this book conceived? When, over pizza and beer with other new students early in my first year of graduate school, somebody dared me to write a term paper on the Epilady personal hair removal device? Or when, digging through some old business journals in order to amuse my beermates with a "gag" term paper, I stumbled onto shocking references to the once-widespread use of x-rays to remove unwanted hair? Or when, after publishing an essay based on that x-ray research, people scattered all over the world—a Nobel Prize–winning biologist in New York, a high school shop teacher in central Oregon, a television producer in London—wrote to me, wanting to learn more? Do these events explain the birth of my interest in hair? Yes, no, perhaps. No matter how many times I am asked, I cannot adequately explain how I came to this book.

Somewhat clearer, however, is why it took me so long to finish it. Challenging emotions—shame, disgust, avoidance—swirled around this project throughout. Not long after I published the essay on x-ray hair removal, I wrote a trusted friend, also a budding academic, to report the encouraging feedback I was receiving on it. "Drop the hair thing, Bec," he replied. "It's stupid." Cowed, I dropped it. Several years and two book projects later, I considered picking the topic back up. Around that time, I happened to be seated next to a famous sociologist during the lunch break of a small professional workshop. He dutifully inquired what I was working on. I replied, with some tentativeness, that I was thinking about pursuing a monograph on body hair. He recoiled perceptibly. "Well, I suppose everyone has to work on *something*," he said, turning his chair away from me abruptly to emphasize the end of our exchange. I spent the rest of the meal in embarrassed silence.

Such comments are trifling, of course. I mention them here because, as all those "personal" questions from readers and listeners suggested, and as conversations with my discerning mother finally compelled me to acknowledge, my own vexed embodiment (embarrassment and all) is intrinsic to this book. To be sure, the point may be extended to other scholarship: as plenty of brilliant work in feminist, queer, disability, and critical race studies has demonstrated, there is no such thing as disembodied, bloodless knowledge, no "view from nowhere." It is only my experience of privilege—the fact that I am usually perceived as a white, straight, able-bodied, middle-class American woman—that allows me to entertain the fantasy that my own body doesn't matter, epistemologically. And yet, while my life history necessarily informs all of my scholarship, only this topic has provoked other people to inquire about the various stakes—emotional, political, physiological—conditioning the research.

So what to say when someone asks me about how I came to this topic? How to acknowledge the bigger truth, that embodiment *does* condition knowledge, without conflating it with my own (not particularly illuminating) experiences with hair? There are no easy answers—only habitable compromises between hope and shame, revelation and discretion, wisdom and absurdity.

NAVIGATING THESE TENSIONS well enough to finish the book required a lot of support. My list of debts is impossibly long. To everyone and everything who helped bring this book to life: thank you.

My first debt is to the students, staff, faculty, and alumni of Bates College, for creating such an exhilarating place to work. The college extended essential funding for this project, not only through my regular salary but also through a Student Research Apprenticeship Award, a Howard Hughes Medical Institute/IDEA Networks of Biomedical Research Excellence Grant, a Charles F. and Evelyn M. Phillips Faculty Fellowship, several other faculty development grants, and an extended sabbatical leave. Additional material support was extended by the Bakken Museum and Library in Minneapolis; the Hartman Center for Sales, Advertising, and Marketing History at Duke University; the Department of the History of Science at Harvard University; the Center for Cultural Studies at the University of California at Santa Cruz; and the Division of the History of Science, Technology, and the Environment at the Royal Institute of Technology, Stockholm. Research for chapter 9 was made possible by a 2008 grant from the National Science Foundation (#0749769, "RNAi,

Race, and the Domestication of Biotechnology: The Emergence of Cosmetic Genomics").

Responses to earlier presentations of this material were wide-ranging, and I appreciate all of the questions and comments offered to me. Warm thanks to audiences at Bates College, Colby College, Columbia University, Drexel University, Harvard University, Illinois College, Maine Women's Policy Center, MIT, the Royal Institute of Technology, the University of California at San Diego, the University of California at Santa Cruz, the University of Maine at Augusta, the University of Maine at Orono, the University of Massachusetts at Amherst, the University of New England, and the University of Pennsylvania. I also received helpful feedback on earlier versions of this work at meetings of the Berkshire Conference on the History of Women, the History of Science Society, the Organization of American Historians, the Society for the History of Technology, the Society for the Social Studies of Science, and the Southern Association for the History of Medicine and Science. Special thanks to the North American Hair Research Society for graciously admitting me as a member. Portions of chapter 3 appeared previously in the *NWSA Journal* (now *Feminist Formations*); portions of chapter 4 previously appeared in *Technology and Culture* and the *Journal of Social History*; portions of chapter 7 appeared in *Australian Feminist Studies*. I thank the Johns Hopkins University Press, Oxford University Press, and Taylor & Francis Group for permission to republish them here.

I also would like to thank Alicia Gilman, Kerry Gross, Perrin Lumbert, and Alison Vander Zanden for their assistance obtaining primary source material; Caelyn Cobb, Ali Desjardin, and Mathieu Duvall for their help obtaining images and permissions; and Denise Begin, Beverly Carter, Jessie Govindasamy, and Lorelei Purrington for their support with last-minute copying, printing, and mailing. Sheila Bodell, Laurie Prendergast, Alexia Traganas, and Emily Wright facilitated the final stages of the book's production. Institutional Review Board protocols forbid me from identifying interview participants by name, but I remain cognizant of their generous offerings of time. For their contributions to this book, I also thank Kiran Asher, Rachel Austin, Myron Beasley, Lisa Botshon, Marisa Brandt, Stephanie Camp, Monica Casper, Monica Chiu, Ryan Conrad, Karen Dearborn, Steven Epstein, Holly Ewing, Michael Fischer, Deborah Fitzgerald, Mats Fridlund, Robert Friedel, Jan Golinski, Robin Hackett, Jennifer Hamilton, Evelynn Hammonds, Donna Haraway, Anne Harrington, Leslie Hill, Monica Hoffman, Sue Houchins, Doug Hubley, Margaret Imber, Lochlann Jain, Emily Kane, Arne Kaijser, Sasha Keller, Sharon Kinsman, Katie Larwa, Nina Lerman, Leo Marx, Lisa Maurizio, Jonathan Metzl, Lisa Jean Moore, Alondra Nelson, Naomi Oreskes, Ronna Pearl, Melinda Plastas, Eve Raimon, Jenny Reardon, Michael Sargent, Chris Schiff, Siobhan Senier, David Serlin, Steven Shapin, Bonnie Shulman, Amy Slaton, John Staudenmaier, Banu Subramaniam, Heidi Taylor, Lynn Thomas, Liz Tobin, Lisa Walker, Harlan Weaver, Debbie Weinstein, Angela Willey, Nina Wormbs, and the anonymous reviewers for this and other presses. Ilene Kalish, Dawn Potter, and Erica Rand all read the whole manuscript, and offered specific suggestions for improvement. My siblings and extended kin offered invaluable cheer and insight. David Barlow transformed me and this project in more ways than I could recount. Beloved Sam helped out by urging me to come play. I am grateful for all.

FINALLY, I EXTEND my deepest thanks to Jill Hopkins Herzig, my mother and treasured intellectual companion. She attuned me to the mystery and beauty of being alive; I, in turn, offer a few lines of dedication in an academic monograph on hair removal. So it goes. I will continue to search for better, more enduring ways to express my love and gratitude—in the meantime, Mom, this book is for you.

Notes

NOTES TO THE INTRODUCTION

1. International Committee of the Red Cross Report, Regional Delegation for United States and Canada (Geoff Loane, Head of Regional Delegation), Washington, DC, February 14, 2007, 26.
2. International Committee of the Red Cross Report, 17.
3. "Inside the Interrogation of Detainee 063," *Time*, Sunday, June 12, 2005, with reporting by Brian Bennett, Timothy J. Burger, Sally B. Donnelly and Viveca Novak, http://www.time.com/time/magazine/article/0,9171,1071284-1,00.html.
4. U.S. Department of Justice, Office of the Inspector General, Oversight and Review Division, "A Review of the FBI's Involvement in and Observations of Detainee Interrogations in Guantanamo Bay, Afghanistan, and Iraq," May 2008, 193.
5. Few English-language commentators criticized the forced removal of detainees' beards. One rare exception juxtaposed a description of the practice with a photograph of a Nazi soldier forcibly shaving a prisoner of war during World War II. See "Our Methods of Being Cruel to Others Are Not as Creative as They Should Be," *Tiny Revolution*, May 27, 2005, http://www.tinyrevolution.com/mt/archives/00529.html. Also see Human Rights Watch Press Release, "U.S.: Religious Humiliation of Muslim Detainees Widespread," *Human Rights Watch*, May 18, 2005, http://www.hrw.org/en/news/2005/05/18/us-religious-humiliation-muslim-detainees-widespread. For a recent example of critics' silence on forced shaving, see Jill Lepore, "The Dark Ages: Terrorism, Counterterrorism, and the Law of Torment," *New Yorker*, March 18, 2013.
6. Rich Lowry, "Close Gitmo?" Tuesday, June 14, 2005, *Townhall.com*, http://townhall.com/columnists/RichLowry/2005/06/14/close_gitmo.

7. "The Guantanamo Bay Controversy," *Hardball with Chris Matthews*, *MSNBC*, June 15, 2005, http://www.msnbc.msn.com/id/8242602.

8. "Stand Firm for Gitmo," *Washington Times*, June 13, 2005, http://washingtontimes.com/news/2005/jun/13/20050613-085444-3748r.

9. Brit Hume, "Discussion of Guantanamo Controversy" (interview with Mara Liasson, Bill Sammon, and Fred Barnes), from *Fox: Special Report*, *Fox News*, June 15, 2005. Transcript accessed through Westlaw's Campus Research, http://campus.westlaw.com.

10. The history of body hair is rather like the history of vibrators in this way. For an elegant discussion of related historiographical issues, see the preface to Rachel P. Maines, *The Technology of Orgasm: "Hysteria," the Vibrator, and Women's Sexual Satisfaction* (Baltimore, MD: Johns Hopkins University Press, 1999).

11. Terence Turner, "The Social Skin," in *Reading the Social Body*, ed. Catherine B. Burroughs and Jeffrey David Ehrenreich (Iowa City: University of Iowa Press, 1993), 18, 38; Sara Ahmed and Jackie Stacey, "Introduction: Dermographies," in *Thinking Through the Skin*, ed. Sara Ahmed and Jackie Stacey (London: Routledge, 2001); Anthony Synnott, *The Body Social: Symbolism, Self, and Society* (London: Routledge, 1993), 103; Jay Prosser, *Second Skins: The Body Narratives of Transsexuality* (New York: Columbia University Press, 1998), esp. 72; Arthur F. Bentley, "The Human Skin: Philosophy's Last Line of Defense," *Philosophy of Science* 8:1 (January 1941): 1–19; Julia Kristeva, *Powers of Horror: An Essay on Abjection* (New York: Columbia University Press, 1982).

12. M. Gregg Bloche and Jonathan H. Marks, "Doctors and Interrogators at Guantanamo Bay," *New England Journal of Medicine*, July 7, 2005; Alfred W. McCoy, *A Question of Torture: CIA Interrogation, from the Cold War to the War on Terror* (New York: Holt, 2006). On the import of classificatory schema more broadly, see Geoffrey C. Bowker and Susan Leigh Star, *Sorting Things Out: Classification and Its Consequences* (Cambridge, MA: MIT Press, 1999).

13. Joan Jacobs Brumberg expertly traces these twined processes in *The Body Project: An Intimate History of American Girls* (New York: Random House, 1997). On shifts in the authority of science and medicine with respect to definitions of suffering, see Rebecca Herzig, *Suffering for Science: Reason and Sacrifice in Modern America* (New Brunswick, NJ: Rutgers University Press, 2005); Keith Wailoo, *Pain: A Political History* (Baltimore, MD: Johns Hopkins University Press, 2014).

14. Adele E. Clarke et al., "Biomedicalization: A Theoretical and Substantive Introduction," in *Biomedicalization: Technoscience, Health, and Illness in the*

U.S., ed. Adele E. Clarke et al. (Durham, NC: Duke University Press, 2010); Jonathan M. Metzl and Anna Kirkland, eds., *Against Health: How Health Became a New Morality* (New York: New York University Press, 2010).

15. Linda A. Bergthold, "Medical Necessity: Do We Need It?" *Health Affairs* 14:4 (1995): 180–90.

16. See, e.g., Michelle O'Brien, "Tracing This Body: Transsexuality, Pharmaceuticals, and Capitalism," in *The Transgender Studies Reader 2*, ed. Susan Stryker and Aren Z. Aizura (New York: Routledge, 2013), 56–65. For further examples of battles over medical need, see C. Michelle Murphy, "The 'Elsewhere within Here' and the MCS Movement," *Configurations* 8:1 (2000): 87–120; Joseph Dumit, "Illnesses You Have to Fight to Get: Facts as Forces in Uncertain, Emergent Illnesses," *Social Science & Medicine* 62:3 (February 2006): 577–90.

17. On the benefits of global perspectives on the history of science, see the related special issue of *Isis* 101:1 (March 2010).

18. Judith Butler, *Precarious Life: The Powers of Mourning and Violence* (London: Verso, 2006), 64.

19. Readers seeking an accessible introduction to current scientific perspectives on skin might consult Nina G. Jablonski, *Skin: A Natural History* (Berkeley: University of California Press, 2006).

20. See Bruno Latour, "On the Partial Existence of Existing and Nonexisting Objects," in *Biographies of Scientific Objects*, ed. Lorraine Daston (Chicago: University of Chicago Press, 2000), 247–69; Sheila Jasanoff, ed., *States of Knowledge: The Co-Production of Science and Social Order* (New York: Routledge, 2004).

21. Londa Schiebinger, "Why Mammals Are Called Mammals," in *Nature's Body: Gender and the Making of Modern Science* (Boston: Beacon, 1993), 40–74.

22. More recently, molecular biologists, drawing on the long-neglected work of the nineteenth-century anatomist Paul Gerson Unna, have wrestled with pluripotent stem cells in the hair follicle: where and how those cells proliferate remain unsettled questions. Interest in hair stem cells is high because they carry none of the political baggage of stem cells derived from human embryos. See P. G. Unna, "Beiträge zur Histologie und Entwicklungsgeschichte der menschlichen Oberhaut und ihrer Anhangsgebilde," *Archiv für mikroskopische Anatomie* 12 (1876): 665–741; George Cotsarelis, "Cutaneous Stem Cells," in *Principles of Tissue Engineering*, ed. Robert Lanza, Robert Langer, and Joseph P. Vacanti (Waltham, MA: Academic Press, 2011); R. J. Morris et al., "Capturing and Profiling Adult Hair Follicle Stem

Cells," *Nature Biotechnology* 22 (2004): 411–17; H. Oshima et al., "Morphogenesis and Renewal of Hair Follicles from Adult Multipotent Stem Cells," *Cell* 104 (2001): 233–45; T. Tumbar et al., "Defining the Epithelial Stem Cell Niche in Skin," *Science* 303 (2004): 359–63; G. Cotsarelis et al., "Label-Retaining Cells Reside in the Bulge Area of Pilosebaceous Unit: Implications for Follicular Stem Cells, Hair Cycle, and Skin Carcinogenesis," *Cell* 61 (1990): 1329–37; Zhicao Yue et al., "Mapping Stem Cell Activities in the Feather Follicle," *Nature*, December 15, 2005, 1026–29.

23. This is not to suggest that only the privileged engage in classifications of the world— merely that I here focus on dominant framings. For a brilliant analysis of the "counterprivileges of biopolitical irrelevance," see Mel Y. Chen, *Animacies: Biopolitics, Racial Mattering, and Queer Affect* (Durham, NC: Duke University Press, 2012), 233.

24. Most of the questions I receive on this front concern male baldness. Interested readers might begin with Burkhard Bilger, "The Power of Hair: Searching for the Next Generation of Baldness Cures," *New Yorker*, January 9, 2006, 43–48; and Julia E. Szymczak and Peter Conrad, "Medicalizing the Aging Male Body: Baldness and Andropause," in *Medicalized Masculinities*, ed. Dana Rosenfeld and Christopher Faircloth (Philadelphia: Temple University Press, 2006), 89–111.

25. Breanne Fahs, "Dreaded 'Otherness': Heteronormative Patrolling in Women's Body Hair Rebellions," *Gender & Society* 25 (2011): 453; Bessie Rigakos, "Women's Attitudes toward Body Hair and Hair Removal: Exploring Racial Differences in Beauty," Wayne State University, Ph.D. dissertation (December 2004), 36; Jeannette Mariscal, "Shave It? Wax It? Leave It? The Bare Truth of Transculturation through the Naked Perspective of Pubic Hair Removal Practices," Bates College, B.A. thesis (May 2012).

26. "Women Spend up to $23,000 to Remove Hair," *UPI.com*, June 24, 2008, http://www.upi.com/Health_News/2008/06/24/Women-spend-up-to-23000-to-remove-hair/UPI-64771214351618; Mure Dickie, Jeremy Grant, Khozen Merchant, and James Politi, "We Can Build a Juggernaut," *Financial Times*, February 4, 2005.

27. Michael Boroughs, Guy Cafri, and J. Thompson, "Male Body Depilation: Prevalence and Associated Features of Body Hair Removal," *Sex Roles* 52:9–10 (May 2005): 637–44. Also see Breanne Fahs, "Shaving It All Off: Examining Social Norms of Body Hair among College Men in a Women's Studies Course," *Women's Studies* 42 (2013): 559–77.

28. See, e.g., Jennifer Finney Boylan, *She's Not There: A Life in Two Genders* (New York: Broadway, 2003), 140; Deirdre McCloskey, *Crossing: A Mem-*

oir (Chicago: University of Chicago Press, 1999), 47; Julie Waters, "The Razor's Edge: Walking the Fine Line of Self," in *Looking Queer: Body Image and Identity in Lesbian, Bisexual, Gay, and Transgender Communities*, ed. Dawn Atkins (New York: Haworth, 1998), 181; Lori Girshick, "Out of Compliance: Masculine-Identified People in Women's Prisons," in *Captive Genders: TransEmbodiment and the Prison Industrial Complex*, ed. Eric A. Stanley and Nat Smith (Edinburgh, Scotland: AK Press, 2011), 189–208.

29. Beyond the United States is another matter, of course. On body hair in other contexts, see Afsaneh Najmabadi, *Women with Mustaches and Men without Beards: Gender and Sexual Anxieties of Iranian Modernity* (Berkeley: University of California Press, 2005); Alf Hiltebeitel and Barbara D. Miller, eds., *Hair: Its Power and Meaning in Asian Cultures* (Albany: State University of New York Press, 1998); Ruth Barcan, *Nudity: A Cultural Anatomy* (Oxford: Berg, 2004); Anne Hollander, *Seeing through Clothes* (Berkeley: University of California Press, 1993); William Ian Miller, *The Anatomy of Disgust* (Cambridge, MA: Harvard University Press, 1997); Howard Eilberg-Schwartz and Wendy Doniger, eds., *Off with Her Head! The Denial of Women's Identity in Myth, Religion, and Culture* (Berkeley: University of California Press, 1995); Larissa Bonfate, "Nudity as a Costume in Classical Art," *American Journal of Archaeology* 93 (1989): 543–70; Margaret R. Miles, *Carnal Knowing: Female Nakedness and Religious Meaning in the Christian West* (Boston: Beacon, 1989); and Virginia Smith, *Clean: A History of Personal Hygiene and Purity* (Oxford: Oxford University Press, 2007).

30. The lengthy legal dispute over the beard of Nidal Hasan, the army psychiatrist sentenced to death for his 2009 shooting spree at Fort Hood, which killed thirteen people and wounded thirty others, points to the particular complexity of military protocol on the matter. See Russell Goldman, "Nidal Hasan's Lawyer to Sue after Army Forcibly Shaves Ft. Hood Shooter," *ABC News*, September 4, 2013.

31. *Ho Ah Kow v. Nunan*, 12 Fed. Cas. 252 (1879); "Secular News," *Christian Observer*, August 3, 1904, 23. On the subjection of masculine-identified people in women's prisons to forced hair removal, see Girshick, "Out of Compliance," 198–99.

32. On the shaving, washing, and oiling of enslaved people's bodies, see Stephanie E. Smallwood, *Saltwater Slavery: A Middle Passage from Africa to American Diaspora* (Cambridge, MA: Harvard University Press, 2007), esp. 160–62. I am grateful to Stephanie Camp for drawing my attention to this phenomenon. Head shaving as a technique of domination also was inflicted on enslaved people, particularly by white women on black women.

Jack Maddox described the wife of a Texas plantation owner punishing "a pretty mulatto girl" by grabbing a pair of scissors and "cropp[ing] that gal's head to the skull"; James Brittian similarly recalled how the "Old Miss" forced his African-born grandmother to wear her hair "shaved to the scalp." See Shane White and Graham White, "Slave Hair and African American Culture in the Eighteenth and Nineteenth Centuries," *Journal of Southern History* 61:1 (February 1995): 68. More recent cases of forced hair removal are recounted in Timothy Williams, "Students Recall Special Schools Run like Jails," *New York Times*, July 24, 2013, A1.

33. Evidence of this cultural aversion may be found in the Planter's "Unibrow" commercial, aired during the 2008 Super Bowl broadcast (see http://www.youtube.com/watch?v=kfzbZJrzo6A). The advertisement presumes that viewers will get the joke: the only possible way a woman with thick, hairy eyebrows might be considered attractive by random men on the street would be (as the commercial reveals) by dousing herself with the scent of Planter's roasted nuts.

34. See, e.g., Carole Cleaver, "A Dirty Story," *Mademoiselle*, April 1958, 46, cited in Suellen Hoy, *Chasing Dirt: The American Pursuit of Cleanliness* (New York: Oxford University Press, 1995), 2.

35. The only two English-language scholarly books on body hair I have found are Alfred F. Niemoeller, *Superfluous Hair and Its Removal* (New York: Harvest House, 1938) and Karín Lesnik-Oberstein, ed., *The Last Taboo: Women and Body Hair* (Manchester, England: Manchester University Press, 2006). The male beard has been the focus of several studies; so, too, have specific cases of "bearded ladies" and other hairy individuals placed on display. The history and politics of black and African American head hair and hairstyling have received far more sustained consideration; that work enables the attention to racialization suffusing this book. Other than that, there has been little scholarly appetite for the history of hair. See Allan Peterkin, *One Thousand Beards: A Cultural History of Facial Hair* (Vancouver, Canada: Arsenal Pulp Press, 2001); Lorraine Daston and Katherine Park, *Wonders and the Order of Nature, 1150–1750* (Cambridge, MA: Zone, 1998); Leslie Fiedler, *Freaks: Myths and Images of the Secret Self* (New York: Simon & Schuster, 1978); Paulette M. Caldwell, "Hair Piece," in *Critical Race Theory*, ed. Richard Delgado (Philadelphia: Temple University Press, 1995), 267–80; Ayana D. Byrd and Lori L. Tharps, *Hair Story: Untangling the Roots of Black Hair in America* (New York: St. Martin's, 2001); Ginetta Candelario, "Hair Race-ing: Dominican Beauty Culture and Identity Production," *Meridians: Feminism, Race, Transnationalism* 1:1 (2000):

128–56; Diane Simon, *Hair: Public, Political, Extremely Personal* (New York: St. Martin's, 2000); Kobena Mercer, "Black Hair/Style Politics," in *Out There: Marginalization and Contemporary Cultures*, ed. Russell Ferguson et al. (New York: New Museum of Contemporary Art, 1992), 247–64; Noliwe M. Rooks, *Hair Raising: Beauty, Culture, and African American Women* (New Brunswick, NJ: Rutgers University Press, 1996); Ashleigh Shelby Rosette and Tracy L. Dumas, "The Hair Dilemma: Conform to Mainstream Expectations or Emphasize Racial Identity?" *Duke Journal of Gender Law and Policy* 14:1 (2007): 407–21; Tracey Owens Patton, "'Hey Girl, Am I More Than My Hair?' African American Women and Their Struggles with Beauty, Body Image, and Hair," *NWSA Journal* 18:2 (Summer 2006): 24–51; Susannah Walker, *Style & Status: Selling Beauty to African American Women, 1920–1975* (Lexington: University Press of Kentucky, 2007); Deborah R. Grayson, "Is It Fake? Black Women's Hair as Spectacle and Spec(tac)ular," *camera obscura* 36 (1995): 13–31; Robyn Anuakan, "'We Real Cool': Beauty, Image, and Style in African-American History," Ph.D dissertation, University of California, Berkeley (2002).

36. There is also a large literature dedicated to explaining hair aversions (and hair fetishes) according to psychoanalytic principles; see chapter 5 below.

37. Nancy Etcoff, *Survival of the Prettiest: The Science of Beauty* (New York: Random House, 1999).

38. James Giles, "Naked Love: The Evolution of Human Hairlessness," *Biological Theory: Integrating Development, Evolution, and Cognition* 5 (1984): 326–36.

39. Mark Pagel and Walter Bodmer, "A Naked Ape Would Have Fewer Parasites," *Proceedings of the Royal Society of London* (Supplement) 270 (2003): S117–19. See also G. G. Schwartz and L. A. Rosenblum, "Allometry of Primate Hair Density and the Evolution of Human Hairlessness," *American Journal of Physical Anthropology* 55:1 (1981): 9–12; Shaoni Bhattacharya, "Early Humans Lost Hair to Beat Bugs," *New Scientist*, June 3, 2003.

40. Ongoing controversy within communities of evolutionary biologists on the matter of humans' relative hairlessness has been a boon to creationists. See, for example, Michael Matthews, "Hairless Hokum," *answersingenesis.org*, August 25, 2003, http://www.answersingenesis.org/articles/2003/08/25/hairless-hokum; "Hairless Apes: Evolution Is Just a Theory," *Debating Christianity and Religion*, http://debatingchristianity.com/forum/viewtopic.php?t=17726; "Another Made-up Story from the *New York Times*: Hair Loss," *evolutionisdead.com*, August 19, 2003, http://www.evolutionisdead.com/darwin.php?did=006.

41. Some writers suggest that pubic and axillary hair must similarly serve an evolutionary purpose, such as carrying pheromones or protecting "the vaginal environment." Note that narratives of "selective pressure" are used both for and against body hair. See, e.g., Liz Porter, "From X-rated to the Everyday: How the Burbs Went Brazilian," *Age*, November 2, 2008, http://www.theage.com.au/action/printArticle?id=253961; Marika Tiggemann and Sarah J. Kenyon, "The Hairlessness Norm: The Removal of Body Hair in Women," *Sex Roles* 39:11–12 (1998): 873–85.

42. Cited in Nicholas Wade, "Why Humans and Their Fur Parted Ways," *New York Times*, August 19, 2003.

43. As Laura Kipnis inimitably writes, "When sociobiologists start shitting in their backyards with dinner guests in the vicinity, maybe their arguments about innateness over culture will start seeming more persuasive." See *Against Love: A Polemic* (New York: Vintage, 2003), 24.

44. On Krao, see Kimberly A. Hamlin, "The 'Case of a Bearded Woman': Hypertrichosis and the Construction of Gender in the Age of Darwin," *American Quarterly* 63:4 (December 2011): 955–81; Lindsey B. Churchill, "What Is It? Difference, Darwin, and the Victorian Freak Show," *Darwin in Atlantic Cultures: Evolutionary Visions of Race, Gender, and Sexuality*, ed. Jeannette Eileen Jones and Patrick B. Sharp (New York: Routledge, 2010), 128–42.

45. This is not to discount the influence of natural selection on hair growth patterns—only to insist, in keeping with my earlier discussion of scientific facts, that our knowledge about hair is inescapably social and historical. The sharp decline in reported cases of pubic lice between 1997 and 2003, a decline attributed by some clinicians to the increased popularity of total genital waxing, suggests the complexity of our evolutionary encounters with nonhuman "companion species" of all kinds. See Suzannah Hills, "Is *Sex and the City* Responsible for the Demise of Pubic Lice?" *Mail Online*, July 4, 2013; Donna J. Haraway, *When Species Meet* (Minneapolis: University of Minnesota Press, 2008).

46. Merran Toerien and Sue Wilkinson, "Gender and Body Hair: Constructing the Feminine Woman," *Women's Studies International Forum* 26:4 (2003): 241; Breanne Fahs and D. A. Delgado, "The Specter of Excess: Race, Class, and Gender in Women's Body Hair Narratives," in *Embodied Resistance: Breaking the Rules, Challenging the Norms*, ed. C. Bobel and S. Kwan (Nashville, TN: Vanderbilt University Press, 2011), 15. See also Susan A. Basow and Amie C. Braman, "Women and Body Hair: Social Perceptions and Attitudes," *Psychology of Women Quarterly* 22:4 (December 1998): 637–45;

Sarah Hildebrandt, "The Last Frontier: Body Norms and Hair Removal Practices in Contemporary American Culture," in *The EmBodyment of American Culture*, ed. Heinz Tschachler et al. (Munich: Lit Verlag, 2003), 59–71; Joan Ferrante, "Biomedical versus Cultural Constructions of Abnormality: The Case of Idiopathic Hirsutism in the United States," *Culture, Medicine, and Psychiatry* 12 (1988): 219–38; Marika Tiggemann and Sarah J. Kenyon, "The Hairlessness Norm: The Removal of Body Hair in Women," *Sex Roles* 39:11–12 (1998): 873–85; Merran Toerien, Sue Wilkinson, and Precilla Y. L. Choi, "Body Hair Removal: The 'Mundane' Production of Normative Femininity," *Sex Roles* 52:5–6 (March 2005): 399–406.

47. Toerien and Wilkinson, "Gender and Body Hair," 333–44; Basow and Braman, "Women and Body Hair," 637–45; Susan A. Basow and J. Willis, "Perceptions of Body Hair on White Women: Effects of Labeling," *Psychological Reports* 89:3 (2001): 571–76.

48. On the influence of consumer capitalism on women's hair removal, see Leonore Riddell, Hannah Varto, and Zoe Hodgson, "Smooth Talking: The Phenomenon of Pubic Hair Removal in Women," *Canadian Journal of Human Sexuality* 19:3 (2010): 129; Marika Tiggemann and Suzanna Hodgson, "The Hairlessness Norm Extended: Reasons for and Predictors of Women's Body Hair Removal at Different Body Sites," *Sex Roles* 59:11 (2008): 895.

49. Marika Tiggemann and Christine Lewis, "Attitudes toward Women's Body Hair: Relationship with Disgust Sensitivity," *Psychology of Women Quarterly* 28:4 (December 2004): 381, 386.

50. Tiggemann and Hodgson, "Hairlessness Norm Extended," 896.

51. David Allyn, *Make Love, Not War: The Sexual Revolution, an Unfettered History* (Boston: Little, Brown, 2000), 285, 287.

52. Naomi Wolf, *The Beauty Myth: How Images of Beauty Are Used against Women* (New York: Morrow, 1991).

53. Tiggemann and Hodgson, "Hairlessness Norm Extended," 890; Tiggemann and Lewis, "Attitudes toward Women's Body Hair," 382; Boroughs et al., "Male Body Depilation."

54. I am influenced here by Thomas Lemke's helpful distinction between bioethical and biopolitical analyses:

Bioethics focuses on the question, what is to be done? It reduces problems to alternatives that can be treated and decided. . . . An analytics of biopolitics, on the other hand, seeks to generate problems. It is interested in questions that have not yet been asked. It raises awareness of all those historical and systematic correlations that regularly remain outside the bioethical framework and its pro-contra debates. . . . As a result, an analytics of biopolitics has a speculative and experimental dimension: it does not affirm what is but anticipates what could be different.

See Thomas Lemke, *Biopolitics: An Advanced Introduction* (New York: New York University Press, 2011), 123. For further discussion of the limitations of such "quandary ethics," see Kwame Anthony Appiah, *Experiments in Ethics* (Cambridge, MA: Harvard University Press, 2008); Anne Pollock, *Medicating Race: Heart Disease and Durable Preoccupations with Difference* (Durham, NC: Duke University Press, 2012), 186.

NOTES TO CHAPTER 1

1. Thomas Jefferson, *Notes on the State of Virginia*, ed. William Peden (Chapel Hill: University of North Carolina Press, 1995), 61. See also Daniel Heath Justice, *Our Fire Survives the Storm: A Cherokee Literary History* (Minneapolis: University of Minnesota Press, 2006), 66; Anthony F. C. Wallace, "Jefferson and the Native Americans," in *Thomas Jefferson and the Changing West*, ed. James P. Ronda (Albuquerque: University of New Mexico Press, 1997), 28.

2. While there were substantial national differences between the various European colonial powers, and equally significant differences between writers on different sides of the Atlantic, I here discuss heterogeneous European and Euro-American sources together as "white." I do so because, as Robert F. Berkhofer explains, "In theory and in practice, each colonizing power, except for Sweden, asserted the same legal power over the persons and territory of Native Americans." However much some U.S. writers sought to distinguish themselves from Europeans, they remained colonizers vis-à-vis Native peoples. See Berkhofer, *The White Man's Indian: Images of the American Indian, from Columbus to the Present* (New York: Knopf, 1978), 119.

3. Scores of white sources report the various depilatory practices observed among "the Indians," yet I have been unable to find any analogous descriptions written by Native authors themselves. This chapter is therefore an analysis of white perceptions. I follow Alexandra Harmon in considering "Indians" as a category established only "in the context of relations with other kinds of people." See Harmon, "Wanted: More Histories of Indian Identity," in *A Companion to American Indian History*, ed. Philip J. Deloria and Neal Salisbury (Malden, MA: Blackwell, 2004), 248; for similar themes, see Rebecca Tsosie, "The New Challenge to Native Identity: An Essay on 'Indigeneity' and 'Whiteness,'" *Washington University Journal of Law and Policy* 4 (2005): 55–98.

4. de Pauw, *Recherches philosophiques sur Les Américains*, vol. 1 (Berlin: Decker, 1772), 39–40.

5. Lewis, writing Tuesday, May 13, 1806, in *The Journals of the Lewis and Clark Expedition*, ed. Gary E. Moulton, vol. 7 (Lincoln: University of Nebraska, 1991 [1814]), 252; Clark echoed the point in his entry of the same day: "[I]n common with other Indian Nations of America they extract their beard, but the men do not uniformly extract the hair below, this is more particularly confined to the females" (254).

6. Alexander de Humboldt [sic], *Political Essay on the Kingdom of New Spain*, trans. John Black, vol. 1 (New York: I. Riley, 1811), 110.

7. Anthony F. C. Wallace, *Jefferson and the Indians: The Tragic Fate of the First Americans* (Cambridge, MA: Belknap Press, 1999), 77; Berkofer, *The White Man's Indian*, 43.

8. William Bartram, *Travels of William Bartram*, ed. Mark Van Doren (New York: Dover, 1955), 26.

9. Londa L. Schiebinger, *Nature's Body: Gender in the Making of Modern Science* (Boston: Beacon, 1993), 123–24.

10. Jefferson bolstered his denunciation of Indian enslavement, for example, by asserting, on the basis of hair, that "nature is the same with them as with the whites." See Jefferson, *Notes*, 61.

11. Justice, *Our Fire*, 60.

12. Berkofer, *The White Man's Indian*, 165; Francis Paul Prucha, ed., *Documents of United States Indian Policy* (Lincoln: University of Nebraska Press, 1989); Mary Hershberger, "Mobilizing Women, Anticipating Abolition: The Struggle against Indian Removal in the 1830s," *Journal of American History* 86:1 (June 1999): 15–40; Maureen Konkle, *Writing Indian Nations: Native Intellectuals and the Politics of Historiography, 1827–1863* (Chapel Hill: University of North Carolina Press, 2004).

13. Tiya Miles, "Removal," in *American Studies: An Anthology*, edited by Janice A. Radway et al. (Chichester, England: Wiley-Blackwell, 2009), 42–43.

14. Lucy Maddox, *Removals: Nineteenth-Century American Literature and the Politics of Indians Affairs* (New York: Oxford University Press, 1991), 10–11; Berkofer, *The White Man's Indian*, 165; and William G. McLoughlin and Walter H. Conser Jr., "'The First Man Was Red': Cherokee Responses to the Debate over Indian Origins, 1760–1860," *American Quarterly* 41:2 (June 1989): 243–64.

15. William Apess, "A Son of the Forest," in *On Our Own Ground: The Complete Writings of William Apess, a Pequot*, ed. Barry O'Connell (Amherst: University of Massachusetts Press, 1992 [1831]), 61.

16. See the classification of mammalia in *A General System of Nature*, trans. William Turton (London: Lackington, Allen, 1806), reproduced in E. Nathaniel Gates, *The Concept of "Race" in Natural and Social Science* (New York: Garland, 1997), 149. On the influence of the Linnaean system on European ideas of race, see Stephen Jay Gould, "The Geometer of Race," *Discover*, November 1994, 67.

17. Buffon, *Natural History, General and Particular*, quoted in Gilbert Chinard, "Eighteenth-Century Theories on America as Human Habitat," *Proceedings of the American Philosophical Society* 91:1 (February 1947): 31. On Buffon, see Robert E. Bieder, *Science Encounters the Indian, 1820–1880* (Norman: University of Oklahoma Press, 1986), 6.

18. Buffon, *Natural History, General and Particular*, quoted in Gilbert Chinard, "Eighteenth-Century Theories," 31.

19. Joyce E. Chaplin, *Subject Matter: Technology, the Body, and Science on the Anglo-American Frontier, 1500–1676* (Cambridge, MA: Harvard University Press, 2001); Stephen J. Gould, "American Polygeny and Craniometry before Darwin: Blacks and Indians as Separate, Inferior Species," in *The "Racial" Economy of Science*, ed. Sandra Harding (Bloomington: Indiana University Press, 1993); Susan Scott Parrish, *American Curiosity: Cultures of Natural History in the Colonial British Atlantic World* (Chapel Hill: University of North Carolina Press, 2006), 78 ff.; Roxann Wheeler, *The Complexion of Race: Categories of Difference in Eighteenth-Century British Culture* (Philadelphia: University of Pennsylvania Press, 2000); Bieder, *Science*; Audrey Smedley, *Race in North America: Origin and Evolution of a Worldview*, 3rd edition (Boulder, CO: Westview, 2007), 90.

20. Edith Snook, "The Beautifying Part of Physic: Women's Cosmetic Practices in Early Modern England," *Journal of Women's History* 20:3 (Fall 2008): 24. See also Parrish, *American Curiosity*, 78 ff.; Wheeler, *Complexion of Race*; Smedley, *Race in North America*, 90; Chandler McC. Brooks, Jerome L. Gilbert, Harold A. Levey, and David R. Curtis, *Humors, Hormones, and Neurosecretions: The Origins and Development of Man's Present Knowledge of the Humoral Control of Body Function* (New York: State University of New York Press, 1962). On the humoral complexities of hairy women, specifically, see Mary E. Fissell, "Hairy Women and Naked Truths: Gender and the Politics of Knowledge in 'Aristotle's Masterpiece,'" *William and Mary Quarterly* 60:1 (January 2003): 43–74.

21. Schiebinger, *Nature's Body*, 120–25; Parrish, *American Curiosity*, 78 ff.; Wheeler, *Complexion of Race*; Allan Peterkin, *One Thousand Beards: A Cul-*

tural History of Facial Hair (Vancouver, Canada: Arsenal Pulp Press, 2001), 33–35.

22. Konkle, *Writing Indian Nations*, 9–10; William Robertson, *History of the Discovery and Settlement of America*, vol. 1 (London: Strahan, 1777), 303, 291.

23. Robertson, *History*, 290.

24. Ibid., 290–91.

25. Ibid.

26. Samuel Stanhope Smith, *An Essay on the Causes of the Variety of Complexion and Figure in the Human Species*, ed. Winthrop Jordan (Cambridge, MA: Belknap Press, 1965 [1787]), 112.

27. Ibid., 191; Bieder, *Science*, 7.

28. Johann Friedrich Blumenbach, "On the Natural Variety of Mankind," in *The Anthropological Treatises of Johann Friedrich Blumenbach*, trans. and ed. Thomas Bendyshe (Boston: Longwood, 1978 [1775]), 224, 129, 127.

29. Ibid., 129.

30. James Cowles Prichard, *The Natural History of Man; Comprising Inquiries into the Modifying Influence of Physical and Moral Agencies on the Different Tribes of the Human Family*, 3rd edition (London: Hippolyte Bailliere, 848), 98.

31. Ibid., 99.

32. Prichard, *Researches into the Physical History of Man*, ed. George W. Stocking (Chicago: University of Chicago Press, 1973 [1813]), 41. On aesthetic preference as a factor in racial variation, see Evelyeen Richards, "Darwin and the Descent of Woman," in *The Wider Domain of Evolutionary Thought*, ed. David Oldroyd and Ian Langham (Dordrecht: Reidel, 1983), 105 n.78.

33. Blumenbach, "Natural Variety of Mankind," 174.

34. Ibid., 173.

35. Knox, cited in Konkle, *Writing Indian Nations*, 15.

36. Konkle, *Writing Indian Nations*, 3; Bieder, *Science*, 9.

37. Hershberger, "Mobilizing Women," 40; Ronald Satz, *American Indian Policy in the Jacksonian Era* (Lincoln: University of Nebraska Press, 1975).

38. Konkle, *Writing Indian Nations*, 5; Bieder, *Science*, 11.

39. The phrase "imperishable" comes from Emerson's discussion of race in "English Traits," in *Selected Writings of Emerson*, ed. Donald McQuade (New York: Modern Library, 1981 [1856]), 523, 525.

40. George Catlin, *Letters and Notes on the Manners, Customs, and Conditions of the North American Indians* (New York: Dover, 1973 [1841–1842]), 2:227.

41. Richard McCausland, "Particulars Relative to the Nature and Customs of the Indians of North-America," *Philosophical Transactions of the Royal Society of London* 76 (1786): 231; Alexander Mackenzie, *Voyages from Montreal through the Continent of North America to the Frozen and Pacific Oceans in 1789 and 1793*, vol. 1 (New York: New Amsterdam Book Company, 1902 [1801]), 234–35; George Juan and Antonio de Ulloa, *A Voyage to South America*, trans. John Adams, vol. 1, 4th edition (London: Stockdale, 1806), 267.

42. Frederic Baraga, *Short History of the North American Indians*, trans. Graham A. MacDonald (Calgary, Canada: University of Calgary Press, 2004 [1837]), 82. Baraga joined a number of other period observers in claiming that Indian men removed their hair in order to paint and tattoo themselves more finely. See, for example, John Heckewelder, *History, Manners, and Customs of the Indian Nations Who Once Inhabited Pennsylvania and the Neighbouring States* (Philadelphia: Historical Society of Pennsylvania, 1876 [1818]), 204; Mark Van Doren, ed., *Travels of William Bartram* (New York: Dover, 1955), 393–94. For further discussion, see Renée L. Bergland, *The National Uncanny: Indian Ghosts and American Subjects* (Lebanon, NH: University Press of New England, 2000), 133–34.

43. "Letter from Eugene Bandel to Augusta Bandel and Julius Bandel, November 22, 1856," in Eugene Bandel, *Frontier Life in the Army, 1854–1861*, trans. Olga Bandel and Richard Jente, ed. Ralph P. Bieber (Glendale, CA: Clark, 1932), 94.

44. Josephine Paterek, *Encyclopedia of American Indian Costume* (Denver: ABC-CLIO, 1994), 21, 231; Edwin Thompson Denig, *The Assiniboine*, edited by J. N. B. Hewitt (Norman: University of Oklahoma Press, 2000), 199.

45. S. S. Haldeman, "Gleanings," *American Antiquarian* 1 (July 1878): 80. Victoria Sherrow, *Encyclopedia of Hair: A Cultural History* (Westport, CT: Greenwood, 2006), 180.

46. McCausland, "Particulars," 230.

47. Heckewelder, *History*, 205.

48. "On the Stature, Form, Colour, &c. of Different Nations," *Boston Magazine*, January 1785, 15; Catlin, *Letters*, 227.

49. The laziness of Indians also was a recurrent theme in formal discussions of Indian policy. See, for instance, Indian Affairs Commissioner William Medill's Annual Report of 1848, excerpted in Prucha, *Documents*, 78. Several readers have asked whether references to scalping were common in white assessments of Indian hair removal; I have found no association between the two practices in period sources.

50. Catlin, *Letters*, 227.

51. Prucha, *Documents*, 80; Wilcomb E. Washburn, *Red Man's Land/White Man's Law: A Study of the Past and Present of the Status of the American Indian* (New York: Scribner's, 1971), 70.

52. "Letter from Ernest De Massey to Marie-Colmbe Arulith de Massey, 1850," in *A Frenchman in the Gold Rush: The Journal of Ernest de Massey, Argonaut of 1849*, trans. Marguerite Eyer Wilbur (San Francisco: California Historical Society, 1927), 60. For more recent expressions of curiosity about Native body hair, see Joseph Boyden, "Bush Country," in *Me Sexy: An Exploration of Native Sex and Sexuality*, ed. Drew Hayden Taylor (Vancouver: Douglas & McIntrye, 2008), 7 ff.

53. Stephanie Pratt, *American Indians in British Art, 1700–1840* (Norman: University of Oklahoma Press, 2005); McLoughlin and Conser, "'The First Man Was Red,'" 252. On relations between debates over Indian removal and abolition, see Nicholas Guyatt, "'The Outskirts of Our Happiness': Race and the Lure of Colonization in the Early Republic," *Journal of American History* 95:4 (March 2009): 986–1011.

54. The phrase "patient examination of facts" is from Samuel George Morton, *An Inquiry into the Distinctive Characteristics of the Aboriginal Race of America*, 2nd edition (Philadelphia: Penington, 1844), 35. On antebellum ethnology, see William Stanton, *The Leopard's Spots: Scientific Attitudes toward Race in America, 1815–1859* (Chicago: University of Chicago Press, 1960); Nancy Stepan, *The Idea of Race in Science: Great Britain, 1800–1900* (Hamden, CT: Archon, 1982); Gates, *The Concept of "Race"*; and Alexandra Cornelius-Diallo, "'I Will Do a Deed for Freedom': Enslaved Women, Proslavery Theorists, and the Contested Discourse of Black Womanhood," in *Shout Out: Women of Color Respond to Violence*, ed. María Ochoa and Barbara K. Ige (Berkeley, CA: Seal Press, 2007), 281–97.

55. See, e.g., "Scientific Items," *National Magazine; Devoted to Literature, Art, and Religion*, July 1854, 96; W. S. Forwood, "The Negro: A Distinct Species, No. 2," *Medical and Surgical Reporter* 11:2 (February 1858): 69–95; "Medical Jurisprudence: A New Physiological Test of Insanity," *American Law Journal* 11:1 (July 1851): 21; "The Heir [Hair] of the Bourbons Determined Physiologically," *Circular* 3:63 (April 29, 1854): 252; "Literature," *Literary World*, June 11, 1853, 471.

56. Peter A. Browne, *The Classification of Mankind, by the Hair and Wool of Their Heads, with the Nomenclature of Human Hybrids* (Philadelphia: Hart, 1852); Peter A. Browne, *Trichologia Mammalium; or, A Treatise on the Organization, Properties, and Uses of Hair and Wool* (Philadelphia: Jones,

1853). These studies were also instrumental to the advent of forensic studies of hair in the 1850s. See Marcelle Lambert and Victor Balthazard, *Le poil de l'homme et des animaux* (Paris: Steinheil, 1910); Gustav Fritsch, *Das Haupthaar und Seine Bildungsstätte Bei Den Rassen Des Menschen* (Berlin: Reimer, 1912–1915); John Glaister, M.D., *A Study of Hairs and Wools Belonging to the Mammalian Group of Animals, including a Special Study of Human Hair, Considered from the Medico-Legal Aspect* (Cairo. Egypt: Misr Press, 1931); K. Lee Lerner and Brenda Wilmoth Lerner, eds., *World of Forensic Science* (Detroit, MI: Thomson Gale, 2006).

57. "Lecture on Hair, Wool, and Sheep Breeding," *The Plough, the Loom, and the Anvil* 4:2 (August 1851): 88–93; "Lecture on Hair, Wool, and Sheep Breeding," *Southern Planter* 11:4 (April 1851): 1–6.

58. See Samuel George Morton, *Crania Americana; or, A Comparative View of the Skulls of Various Aboriginal Nations of North and South America, to Which Is Prefixed an Essay on the Varieties of the Human Species* (Philadelphia: Dobson, 1839), reprinted by Robert Bernasconi, ed. (Bristol, England: Thoemmes, 2002). Comparative racial measurements of hair were particularly popular in French anthropology. See, for instance, Paul Broca, *Atlas d'anatomie Descriptive du Corps Humain* (Paris: Masson, 1879), 37, cited in Robert V. Guthrie, *Even the Rat Was White: A Historical View of Psychology*, 2nd edition (Boston: Allyn and Bacon, 1998), 17; Paul Topinard, *Anthropology* (London: Chapman and Hall, 1894); M. Pruner-Bey, "De la chevelure comme caractáistique des races humaines d'aprés des recherches microscopiques," *Mémoires, Societé Anthropologique de Paris* ser. 1, vol. 2 (1865): 1–35; M. Pruner-Bey, "Deuxième serie d'observations microscopiques sur la chevelure," *Mémoires, Société d'Anthropologie de Paris* ser. 1, vol. 3 (1868): 77–98; J. Denniker, "Essai d'un classification des races humaines, basee uniquement sur les caracteres physiques," *Bulletins, Societe d'Anthropologie de Paris*, ser. 3, vol. 12 (1889): 320–36. For a thorough review of the anthropometric literature, see Mildred Trotter, "A Review of the Classifications of Hair," *American Journal of Physical Anthropology* 24:1 (July–September 1938): 105–26.

59. See Michael Pettit, "Joseph Jastrow, the Psychology of Deception, and the Racial Economy of Observation," *Journal of the History of the Behavioral Sciences* 43:2 (Spring 2007): 162; Evelynn M. Hammonds and Rebecca M. Herzig, *The Nature of Difference: Sciences of Race in the United States from Jefferson to Genomics* (Cambridge, MA: MIT Press, 2009).

60. Charles J. Stillé, *History of the United States Sanitary Commission; Being the General Report of Its Work during the War of the Rebellion* (Philadel-

phia: Lippincott, 1866), 460.

61. Lundy Braun, "Spirometry, Measurement, and Race in the Nineteenth Century," *Journal of the History of Medicine and Allied Sciences* 60:2 (April 2005): 148. See also Haller, "Race, Mortality, and Life Insurance," *Journal of the History of Medicine and Allied Sciences* 25 (1970): 247–61.

62. Benjamin Apthorp Gould, *Investigations in the Military and Anthropological Statistics of American Soldiers* (New York: Hurd and Houghton, 1869), 568. See also J. H. Baxter, *Statistics, Medical and Anthropological, of the Provost Marshal-General's Bureau, Derived from Records of the Examination for Military Service in the Armies of the United States during the Late War of the Rebellion, of over a Million Recruits, Drafted Men, Substitutes, and Enrolled Men*, 2 vols. (Washington, DC: Government Printing Office, 1875), 1:61; Arthur Riss, *Race, Slavery, and Liberalism in Nineteenth-Century American Literature* (New York: Cambridge University Press, 2006), 102.

63. Gould, *Investigations*, 568.

64. Ibid., 569.

65. See Baxter, *Statistics, Medical and Anthropological*, 1:61; Riss, *Race*, 102; Braun, "Spirometry," 148; Haller, "Race," 247–61.

NOTES TO CHAPTER 2

1. Kathy Peiss, *Hope in a Jar: The Making of America's Beauty Culture* (New York: Metropolitan, 1998), 15; Maggie Angeloglou, *A History of Make-Up* (London: Macmillan, 1970), 75–76; Lois W. Banner, *American Beauty* (Chicago: University of Chicago Press, 1983), 42, 51.

2. The custom of covering the female body with clothing necessarily put emphasis on the face. If it were "the fashion to go naked," Lady Mary Wortley Montagu mused at the time, "the face would be hardly observed." See *Letters from Egypt* (London: Virago, 1983 [1865]), 59.

3. Nell Irvin Painter, "The White Beauty Ideal as Science," in *The History of White People* (New York: Norton, 2010), 67, 70; Melissa Percival, "Introduction," in Melissa Percival and Graeme Tytler, eds., *Physiognomy in Profile: Lavater's Impact on European Culture* (Newark: University of Delaware Press, 2005), 20, 17; Lucy Hartley, *Physiognomy and the Meaning of Expression in Nineteenth-Century Culture* (Cambridge: Cambridge University Press, 2001); Graeme Tytler, *Physiognomy in the European Novel: Faces and Fortunes* (Princeton, NJ: Princeton University Press, 1982).

4. See, e.g., Jane Sharp, *The Midwives Book; or The Whole Art of Midwifery Discovered*, ed. Elaine Hobby (New York: Oxford University Press, 2009

[1671]), 287.

5. Ellen van Oost, "Materialized Gender: How Shavers Configure the Users' Femininity and Masculinity," in *How Users Matter: The Co-Construction of Users and Technologies*, ed. Nelly Oudshoorn and Trevor Pinch (Cambridge, MA: MIT Press, 2003), 197. Herman Melville deftly explored the complex relations between slaveholding whites and black "body-servants" skilled with the use of cut-throat razors in the pivotal shaving scene of his 1855 novella, *Benito Cereno*. On the novella's indebtedness to ongoing ethnological debates over racial origins, see Allan Moore Emery, "The Topicality of Depravity in 'Benito Cereno,'" *American Literature* 55:3 (October 1983): 316–31.

6. "Transmission of Syphilis through Shaving," *Medical and Surgical Reporter* 63:6 (August 1890): 166.

7. On the history of barbering, see Allan D. Peterkin, *One Thousand Beards: A Cultural History of Facial Hair* (Vancouver, Canada: Arsenal Pulp Press, 2001), 69–73; Banner, *American Beauty*, 36–37.

8. See, e.g., "Barbers—Ancient and Modern," *Saturday Evening Post*, February 1875, 4; Paul Starr, *The Social Transformation of American Medicine: The Rise of a Sovereign Profession and the Making of a Vast Industry* (New York: Basic Books, 1982), 37–38; Celeste Chamberland, "Honor, Brotherhood, and the Corporate Ethos of London's Barber-Surgeons' Company, 1570–1640," *Journal of the History of Medicine and Allied Sciences* 64:3 (July 2009): 300–332; Mary Roth Walsh, *"Doctors Wanted: No Women Need Apply": Sexual Barriers in the Medical Profession, 1835–1975* (New Haven, CT: Yale University Press, 1977); Lillian R. Furst, ed., *Women Healers and Physicians: Climbing a Long Hill* (Lexington: University Press of Kentucky, 1997); Margaret Pelling, "Appearance and Reality: Barber-Surgeons, the Body, and Disease," in A. L. Beier and Roger Finlay, eds., *London, 1500–1800: The Making of the Metropolis* (London: Longman, 1985), 82–112; Rebecca J. Tannenbaum, *The Healer's Calling: Women and Medicine in Early New England* (Ithaca, NY: Cornell University Press, 2002).

9. See Edith Snook, "The Beautifying Part of Physic: Women's Cosmetic Practices in Early Modern England," *Journal of Women's History* 20:3 (Fall 2008): 12. Also see Peiss, *Hope in a Jar*, 15; Angeloglou, *A History of Make-Up*, 75–76; Banner, *American Beauty*, 42, 51; Neville Williams, *Powder and Paint: A History of the Englishwoman's Toilet, Elizabeth I–Elizabeth II* (London: Longmans, Green, 1957), 44.

10. Eucharius Rösslin, *The Birth of Mankind: Otherwise Named, The Woman's Book*, ed. Elaine Hobby (Surrey, England: Ashgate, 2009), 199.

11. Cited in C. Henri Leonard, *The Hair: Its Growth, Care, Diseases, and Treat-*

ment (Detroit: C. Henri Leonard, Medical Book Publisher, 1880), 106–7.

12. Bethel Solomons, "Disorders of the Hair and Their Treatment before the 18ᵗʰ Century," *British Journal of Dermatology* 78:2 (1966): 115.

13. Johann Jacob Wecker, *Cosmeticks: or, The Beautifying Part of Physick* (London: Printed by Thomas Johnson, 1660), 70–77.

14. Peterkin, *One Thousand Beards*, 106; Williams, *Powder and Paint*, 44.

15. Peiss, *Hope in a Jar*, 13; Herbert C. Covey, *African American Slave Medicine: Herbal and Non-Herbal Treatments* (Lanham, MD: Lexington, 2007).

16. Philosopher Andrew Ure acknowledged this skill. See *A Dictionary of Arts, Manufactures, and Mines; Containing a Clear Exposition of Their Principles and Practice* (New York: Appleton, 1847), 393.

17. As recently as 2005, physicians in Japan reported that a 49-year-old woman, following a recipe for homemade depilatories reported on a popular television program, was seriously injured when her compound of soymilk, lemon, and absolute ethanol combusted on the stove. See Yasunori Yamamoto et al., "Burns in the Homemade Process of Depilatory Lotion Introduced by a Popular TV Program," *Nessho* 31:3 (2005): 169–74.

18. Peiss, *Hope in a Jar*, 12–13; Covey, *African American Slave Medicine*; Sharla M. Fett, *Working Cures: Healing, Health, and Power on Southern Slave Plantations* (Chapel Hill: University of North Carolina Press, 2002), 63. On the gendering of herbal knowledge, see Susan E. Klepp, "Lost, Hidden, Obstructed, and Repressed: Contraceptive and Abortive Technology in the Early Delaware Valley," in *Early American Technology*, 83–89; Edward Shorter, *A History of Women's Bodies* (New York: Basic Books, 1982), 179–83; Linda Gordon, *The Moral Property of Women: A History of Birth Control Politics in America* (Urbana: University of Illinois Press, 2002), 16; James C. Mohr, *Abortion in America: The Origins and Evolutions of National Policy, 1800–1900* (New York: Oxford University Press, 1978), 6–14; Williams, *Powder and Paint*, 44; Rebecca Laroche, *Medical Authority and Englishwomen's Herbal Texts, 1550–1650* (Burlington, VT: Ashgate, 2009).

19. The process of making pins for sewing, for instance, was specialized in Britain (where as many as seventeen people, each completing a small task, worked on each pin) but automated in the United States (which relied on machines that completed most of the operations automatically). See Brooke Hindle and Steven Lubar, *Engines of Change: The American Industrial Revolution, 1790–1860* (Washington, DC: Smithsonian Institution Press, 1986), 153.

20. Walter Licht, *Industrializing America: The Nineteenth Century* (Baltimore, MD: Johns Hopkins University Press, 1995), 38; Hindle and Lubar,

Engines of Change, 185; Philip Scranton, *Proprietary Capitalism: The Textile Manufacture at Philadelphia, 1800–1885* (Cambridge: Cambridge University Press, 1983); Michael Brewster Folsom and Steven D. Lubar, eds., *The Philosophy of Manufactures: Early Debates over Industrialization in the United States* (Cambridge, MA: MIT Press, 1982).

21. Barbara Ehrenreich and Deirdre English, "Microbes and the Manufacture of Housework," *For Her Own Good: 150 Years of the Experts' Advice to Women* (Garden City, NY: Anchor Press/Doubleday, 1978); Ann Oakley, *Woman's Work: The Housewife Past and Present* (New York: Vintage, 1976); Eleanor Flexner, *Century of Struggle: The Women's Rights Movement in America* (New York: New Viewpoints, 1975); Ruth Schwartz Cowan, *More Work for Mother: The Ironies of Household Technology from the Open Hearth to the Microwave* (New York: Basic Books, 1983).

22. Elizabeth Mendall, "Singular Advertisement," *Philadelphia Repository and Weekly Register,* November 21, 1801, 2.

23. Banner, *American Beauty,* 40; *The Museum of Foreign Literature, Science, and Art* [Philadelphia], April 1, 1823, 314–29; "Perfumery at Wholesale," *Workingman's Advocate,* August 4, 1832, 3; *Maine Farmer* [Augusta], November 7, 1844, 3. Advertising copy suggests that women were the intended users of these products, a fact affirmed by journalists' assertions that razors alone were powerful enough for masculine faces, their beards being "far too stubborn to yield to anything but the daily attacks of the sheer steel." "Thoughts on Beards," *Blackwood's Edinburgh Review,* October 1833, 676. See also "Gouraud's Library of Romance," *Subterranean,* December 20, 1845; "Dr. F. Felix Gouraud's Poudres Subtiles for Eradicating Human Superfluous Hair," *New World,* June 11, 1842, 386.

24. Robert Bentley Todd, ed., *The Cyclopaedia of Anatomy and Physiology,* vol. 4 (London: Longman, Brown, Green, Longmans, & Roberts, 1835–59), 169.

25. James Harvey Young, "Patent Medicines: An Early Example of Competitive Marketing," *Journal of Economic History* 20:4 (December 1960): 656.

26. Ann Anderson, *Snake Oil, Hustlers, and Hambones: The American Medicine Show* (Jefferson: McFarland, 2000); James Harvey Young, *The Toadstool Millionaires: A Social History of Patent Medicines in America before Federal Regulation* (Princeton, NJ: Princeton University Press, 1961); S. Stander, "Transatlantic Trade in Pharmaceuticals during the Industrial Revolution," *Bulletin of the History of Medicine* 43:4 (July/August 1969): 326–43; Joseph W. England, ed., *The First Century of the Philadelphia College of Pharmacy* (Philadelphia: Philadelphia College of Pharmacy and Science, 1922); A. C. Cantley, "Some Facts about Making Patent Medicines," *Chau-*

tauquan 27 (1898): 387–90. Terms and categories such as "perfumer" or "barber" were themselves elastic. See John Strachan, *Advertising and Satirical Culture in the Romantic Period* (Cambridge: Cambridge University Press, 2007), 204; Peiss, *Hope in a Jar,* 19–20.

27. Young, "Patent Medicines," 652.

28. Cantley, "Some Facts," 388; Mary P. Ryan, *Mysteries of Sex: Tracing Women and Men through American History* (Chapel Hill: University of North Carolina Press, 2006), 83. On the role of the nineteenth-century proprietary medicine industry in the rise of professional advertising and business methods more generally, see Jackson Lears, *Fables of Abundance: A Cultural History of Advertising in America* (New York: Basic Books, 1994), esp. 88–99; Pamela Laird, *Advertising Progress: American Business and the Rise of Consumer Marketing* (Baltimore, MD: Johns Hopkins University Press, 1998).

29. Steve Edwards, "Factory and Fantasy in Andrew Ure," *Journal of Design History* 14:1 (2001): 20.

30. Strachan, *Advertising,* 65; John Rudolphy, *Chemical and Pharmaceutical Directory of All the Chemicals and Preparations (Compound Drugs) Now in General Use in the Drug Trade* (Chicago: John Rudolphy, 1877), 30.

31. Advertisement, *New England Galaxy and Masonic Magazine,* November 13, 1818, 17; Ryland W. Greene, *Lippincott's Medical Dictionary* (Philadelphia: Lippincott, 1906), 99.

32. "Atkinson's Depilatory," *Liberator,* October 23, 1840, 171. Roughly three-quarters of the *Liberator*'s subscribers were black. See C. Peter Ripley, *The Black Abolitionist Papers.* Vol. 3, *The United States, 1830–1846* (Chapel Hill: University of North Carolina Press, 1991), 9.

33. Advertisement, *New England Galaxy and United States Literary Advertiser,* August 1, 1831, 3.

34. Banner, *American Beauty,* 40.

35. See Ishbel Ross, *Crusades and Crinolines: The Life and Times of Ellen Curtis Demorest and William Jennings Demorest* (New York: Harper & Row, 1963); Beverly Lowry, *Her Dream of Dreams: The Rise and Triumph of Madam C. J. Walker* (New York: Knopf, 2003); A'Lelia Bundles, *On Her Own Ground: The Life and Times of Madam C. J. Walker* (New York: Scribner, 2001); and Lindy Woodhead, *War Paint: Madame Helena Rubinstein and Miss Elizabeth Arden: Their Lives, Their Times, Their Rivalry* (Hoboken, NJ: Wiley, 2003).

36. The situation appeared somewhat different in Europe, for reasons that are unclear. In 1860, American newspapers reported the legal troubles of a Pa-

risian businesswoman known as Madame Chantal (née Biche), whose celebrated "Eau Indienne Chantal" liquid depilatory not only failed to remove
hair but also "caused a painful wound and disagreeable eruption." Biche
was sentenced to six days in prison. See "News Items," *Saturday Evening
Post*, June 9, 1860, 7.

37. Garrick E. Louis, "A Historical Context of Municipal Solid Waste Management in the United States," *Waste Management and Research* 22 (2004):
307.

38. William Cronon, *Nature's Metropolis: Chicago and the Great West* (New
York: Norton, 1991), 225; Siegfried Giedion, *Mechanization Takes Com-
mand: A Contribution to Anonymous History* (New York: Oxford University
Press, 1948), 216–18; Richard G. Arms, "From Disassembly to Assembly:
Cincinnati; The Birthplace of Mass-Production," *Bulletin of the Historical
and Philosophical Society of Cincinnati* 17 (1959): 195–203.

39. Edward Andrew Parnell, *Applied Chemistry: In Manufactures, Arts, and
Domestic Economy* (New York: Appleton, 1844), 124.

40. Siegfried Giedion, "Mechanization and Death: Meat," *Mechanization
Takes Command* (New York: Norton, 1948), 209–46.

41. Ure, *Dictionary of Arts.* On Ure's influence, see R.J.F., "Ure's Dictionary
of Arts," *Nature*, July 8, 1875, 182; Edwards, "Factory and Fantasy," 17–33;
William H. Brock, *The Chemical Tree: A History of Chemistry* (New York:
Norton, 2000), 272.

42. The first U.S. patent for a chemical depilatory—potash combined with
steam—appears to have been granted on May 15, 1841. (Earlier patents
protected the use of steam in lieu of "water, acids, or other materials" to
remove "wool and hair from skins.") On antebellum chemical arts, see
Agnes Hannay, "A Chronicle of Industry on the Mill River," *Smith College Studies in History* 21:1–4 (October 1935–July 1936): 27–29; J. Leander
Bishop, *A History of American Manufactures from 1608 to 1860* (Philadelphia: Young, 1868); Susan Banson, "Women and the Family Economy in
the Early Republic: The Case of Elizabeth Meredith," *Journal of the Early
Republic* 16:1 (Spring 1996): 47–71; Trevor Harvey Levere, *Transforming
Matter: A History of Chemistry from Alchemy to the Buckball* (Baltimore.
MD: Johns Hopkins University Press, 2001), chap. 4; Brock, *Chemical Tree*,
chap. 8; Ursula Klein, "Two Cultures of Organic Chemistry in the Nine-
teenth Century: A Structural Comparison," in *Experiments, Models, Paper
Tools: Cultures of Organic Chemistry in the Nineteenth Century* (Stanford,
CA: Stanford University Press, 2003).

43. Theodore Steinberg, *Nature Incorporated: Industrialization and the Waters*

of New England (Cambridge: Cambridge University Press, 1991), esp. 211; Cronon, *Nature's Metropolis*, esp. 228; Palanisamy Thankikaivelan et al., "Recent Trends in Leather Making: Processes, Problems, and Pathways," *Critical Reviews in Environmental Science and Technology* 35 (2005): 37–79.

44. Thomas Greene Fessenden, "Political Economy," *New England Farmer*, March 2, 1831, 257.

45. Similarly, people who developed expertise in the manufacture of medicinal or cosmetic chemicals could turn the same skills toward agricultural or industrial ends. See Joseph W. England, ed., *The First Century of the Philadelphia College of Pharmacy, 1821–1921* (Philadelphia: Philadelphia College of Pharmacy and Science, 1922), esp. 35 ff.

46. G. W. Septimus Piesse, *The Art of Perfumery, and Method of Obtaining the Odors of Plants* (Philadelphia: Lindsay and Blakiston, 1857), 232–33.

47. I found no expressions of concern in the period regarding the effects of caustic hair removers on tannery *workers*, despite the fact that they employed massive numbers of people (one antebellum tanner alone, a facility in New York State, employed thirty thousand men during its twenty years of operation. See Bishop, *History of American Manufactures*, 681). A 1934 discussion of chemical depilatories noted that tannery workers "frequently suffer skin damage" from contact with the sulfides used for dehairing hides. See M. C. Phillips, *Skin Deep: The Truth about Beauty Aids—Safe and Harmful* (New York: Vanguard, 1934), 93, 97, 99.

48. See, e.g., Albert H. Stone's patent for a "Depilatory, and process of making it" [No. 732,323], United States Patent Office (June 30, 1903).

49. On similar problems facing users of patent medicines, see Fran Hawthorne, *Inside the FDA: The Business and Politics behind the Drugs We Take and the Food We Eat* (Hoboken, NJ: Wiley, 2005), 36. I use the word "purchaser" here rather than "consumer," since many of the purchasers here probably knew the clerks and druggists from whom they obtained early depilatories; the truly complex, anonymous systems of production and distribution that characterize mass consumption were in their infancy. I am influenced on this point by Susan Strasser's discussion in *Waste and Want: A Social History of Trash* (New York: Metropolitan, 1999), 170–71.

50. Tabitha Toilet, "Amusing," *Boston Weekly Magazine*, May 26, 1804, 122.

51. "Useful Receipts," *Saturday Evening Post*, July 19, 1856, 4.

52. "Superfluous Hair," *Lady's Book*, April 1831, 192; "Superfluous Hair," *Journal of Health*, January 12, 1831, 137.

53. "Cosmetics and Cosmetic Survey," *Medical and Surgical Reporter*, Febru-

ary 5, 1870, 116.

54. Gwen Kay, "Healthy Public Relations: The FDA's 1930s Legislative Campaign," *Bulletin of the History of Medicine* 75:3 (2001): 446–87; Gustavus A. Weber, *The Food, Drug, and Insecticide Administration: Its History, Activities, and Organization* (Baltimore, MD: Johns Hopkins University Press, 1928), esp. chap. 1; John P. Swann, "Food and Drug Administration," in *A Historical Guide to the U.S. Government*, ed. George Thomas Kurian (New York: Oxford University Press, 1998), 252; Hawthorne, *Inside the FDA*, 36; Philips J. Hilts, *Protecting America's Health: The FDA, Business, and One Hundred Years of Regulation* (New York: Knopf, 2003).

55. Banner, *American Beauty*, 43; Deborah A. Sullivan, *Cosmetic Surgery: The Cutting Edge of Commercial Medicine in America* (New Brunswick, NJ: Rutgers University Press, 2001), 156; Kathleen Endres, "Introduction," in *Women's Periodicals in the United States: Consumer Magazines*, ed. Kathleen Endres and Therese Lueck (Westport, CT: Greenwood, 1995); Barbara Welter, "The Cult of True Womanhood, 1820–1860," in *The Underside of American History: Other Readings*, ed. Thomas R. Frazier (New York: Harcourt Brace Jovanovich, 1973).

56. Advertisement, *New England Galaxy and United States Literary Advertiser*, August 1, 1831, 3; "Depilatory" [advertisement], *New England Galaxy and United States Literary Advertiser*, December 8, 1832, 4.

57. [Richard] Edwards and [?] Critten, eds., *New York's Great Industries* (New York: Historical Publishing Company, 1885), 180; Hazel Elizabeth Putnam, *Bottled before 1865* (Los Angeles: Rapid Blue Print, 1968). Price conversions are based on the percentage increase in the Consumer Price Index from 1839 to 2013.

58. Jon Miller and David Muir, *The Business of Brands* (Chichester, England: Wiley, 2004), 4, xi; Naomi Klein, *No Logo: Taking Aim at the Brand Bullies* (New York: Picador, 1999), 6; "The Right to a Name: Peculiar Suit Begun by 'Dr.' Gouraud's Disinherited Son," *New York Times*, June 22, 1886; *New York Times*, July 4, 1853, 4; Isidor Neumann, *Handbook of Skin Diseases*, trans. Lucius D. Bulkley (New York: Appleton, 1872), 284; Banner, *American Beauty*, 44; "Right to a Name," *New York Times*. See also Edwards and Critten, *New York's Great Industries*, 180.

59. Victoria Sherrow, *For Appearance' Sake: The Historical Encyclopedia of Good Looks, Beauty, and Grooming* (Phoenix, AZ: Oryx, 2001), 53; Peterkin, *One Thousand Beards*, 106; Banner, *American Beauty*, 44.

60. Gérard de Nerval, *Journey to the Orient*, trans. N. Glass (London: M. Haag, 1984 [1851]); Edward W. Said, *Orientalism* (New York: Vintage,

1979 [1978]), esp. 180–84; E. Littmann, ed., "The Legend of the Queen of Sheba," in *Bibliotheca Abessinica: Studies concerning the Languages, Literature, and History of Abyssinia* (Leyden: Brill, 1904), 32. Jacob Lassner traces various retellings of the queen's story in *Demonizing the Queen of Sheba: Boundaries of Gender and Culture in Postbiblical Judaism and Medieval Islam* (Chicago: University of Chicago Press, 1993); on her use of depilatories, see page 20.

61. Sarah Berry, *Screen Style: Fashion and Femininity in 1930s Hollywood* (Minneapolis: University of Minnesota Press, 2000), 132. See also Aileen Ribeiro, *Facing Beauty: Painted Women and Cosmetic Art* (New Haven, CT: Yale University Press, 2011), 170.

62. Jack Kelly, "Kill the Pirates," *Pittsburgh Post-Gazette*, April 12, 2009; Joshua E. London, *Victory in Tripoli: How America's War with the Barbary Pirates Established the U.S. Navy and Shaped a Nation* (Hoboken, NJ: Wiley, 2005); Richard Zacks, *The Pirate Coast: Thomas Jefferson, the First Marines, and the Secret Mission of 1805* (New York: Hyperion, 2005); Robert J. Allison, *The Crescent Obscured: The United States and the Muslim World, 1776–1815* (New York: Oxford University Press, 1995), xv, 17.

63. European women had access to "mysterious" women's spaces that male travelers did not; their resulting preoccupations with harem and bath took somewhat different forms. See Shirley Foster, "Colonialism and Gender in the East: Representations of the Harem in the Writings of Women Travellers," *Yearbook of English Studies* 34 (2004): 6–17; Mary Roberts, *Intimate Outsiders: The Harem in Ottoman and Orientalist Art and Travel Literature* (Durham, NC: Duke University Press, 2007); M. S. Anderson, *The Eastern Question* (London: Macmillan, 1966).

64. Nah'nah Kulsūm, *Customs and Manners of the Women of Persia*, trans. James Atkinson (London: Cox, 1832), vi.

65. Kulsūm, *Customs*, 17–18. I have been unable to determine whether the Orientalist Atkinson is related to the famous proprietor of depilatories. See, for instance, J. Ruhrach, "James Atkinson and His Medical Bibliography," *Annals of Medical History* 6 (1924): 200–221; H. Rolleston, "The Two James Atkinsons: James Atkinson of York (1759–1839), James Atkinson, the Persian Scholar (1780–1852)," *Annals of Medical History* 3rd ser., 3 (1941): 175–82.

66. Richard Burton, *Arabian Nights*, vol. 4 (Lawrence, KS: Digireads.com, 2008), 255–56; Edward William Lane, *An Account of the Manners and Customs of the Modern Egyptians* (London: John Murray, 1860 [1836]), 343, 41; Alexander Russell, *Natural History of Aleppo* (London: A. Millar, 1856), 86;

Erasmus Wilson, *The Eastern, or Turkish Bath; Its History* (London: John Churchill, 1861).

67. "On Bathing: No. 10, Vapour Bath," *The Casket: Consisting of Literary, Entertaining, and Instructive Tales, Original Essays, Delineations of Character . . .* , vol. 1 (London: Cowie and Strange, 1828) [reprinted from *The Casket*, September 22, 1827, 269].

68. Ure, *Dictionary of Arts*, 393.

69. Sarah Cheang, "Selling China: Class, Gender, and Orientalism at the Department Store," *Journal of Design History* 20:1 (2007): 2; Erika Rappaport, *Shopping for Pleasure: Women in the Making of London's West End* (Princeton, NJ: Princeton University Press, 2000), 21, 32; William Leach, *Land of Desire: Merchants, Power, and the Rise of a New American Culture* (New York: Pantheon, 1993).

70. Scholars of nineteenth-century Orientalism have shown how women's domestic practices served as crucial points of contact between colonizer and colonized; changing customs of hair removal might well be seen in the same light: as a "contact zone" between domestic and industrial spheres. See, e.g., Cheang, "Selling China," 3; Joanna de Groot, "'Sex' and 'Race': The Construction of Language and Image in the Nineteenth Century," in *Cultures of Empire: A Reader*, ed. Catherine Hall (New York: Routledge, 2000), 37–60; Reina Lewis, *Gendering Orientalism: Race, Femininity, and Representation* (London: Routledge, 1996); Ann Laura Stoler, *Carnal Knowledge and Imperial Power: Race and the Intimate in Colonial Rule* (Berkeley: University of California Press, 2002); Mary Louise Pratt, *Imperial Eyes: Travel Writing and Transculturation* (New York: Routledge, 1992); Anne McClintock, *Imperial Leather: Race, Gender, and Sexuality in the Colonial Contest* (New York: Routledge, 1995). The Orientalist themes apparent in these products predate by several decades the fashion for "mosques, temples, and desert oases" that took off in American merchandising in the 1890s. See Leach, *Land of Desire*, 104.

71. "National Tastes and Antipathies," *Workingman's Advocate*, October 16, 1830, 2.

72. "Literary Notices," *Ladies' Magazine and Literary Gazette*, April 1833, 185.

73. *The Toilette of Health, Beauty, and Fashion* (Boston: Allen and Ticknor, 1834), 52.

74. Ure, *Dictionary of Arts*, 393.

75. Samuel P. Hays, *The Response to Industrialization: 1885–1914* (Chicago: University of Chicago Press, 1957), 15; Laurel Thatcher Ulrich, *The Age of*

Homespun: Objects and Stories in the Creation of an American Myth (New York: Knopf, 2001), 414.

NOTES TO CHAPTER 3

1. "Mummies," *Littell's Living Age*, December 6, 1862, 471.
2. Charles Darwin, *The Descent of Man, and Selection in Relation to Sex* (Princeton, NJ: Princeton University Press, 1981 [1871]), 2–3.
3. Rebecca Stott, *Darwin's Ghosts: The Secret History of Evolution* (New York: Spiegel & Grau, 2012); Peter Bowler, *The Eclipse of Darwinism* (Baltimore, MD: Johns Hopkins University Press, 1983); Nancy Stepan, *The Idea of Race and Science: Great Britain, 1800–1960* (New York: Macmillan, 1982), 61–62; Bernard Grant Campbell, ed., *Sexual Selection and the Descent of Man, 1871–1971* (Chicago: Aldine, 1972).
4. Darwin, *Descent of Man*, 340, 349, 348.
5. George Catlin, *Letters and Notes on the Manners, Customs, and Conditions of the North American Indians* (New York: Dover, 1973 [1841-1842]; Benjamin Apthorp Gould, *Investigations in the Military and Anthropological Statistics of American Soldiers* (New York: Hurd and Houghton, 1869), On Gould's influence on Darwin, see Lundy Braun, "Spirometry, Measurement, and Race in the Nineteenth Century," *Journal of the History of Medicine and Allied Sciences* 60:2 (April 2005): 158.
6. Darwin, *Descent of Man*, 361.
7. Ibid., 375.
8. Ibid., 376.
9. Ibid., 375.
10. Ibid., 376.
11. Darwin to A. R. Wallace (March 16, 1871), in *The Life and Letters of Charles Darwin*, vol. 2 (New York: Appleton, 1888), 317.
12. Darwin, *Descent of Man*, 338.
13. Ibid., 384. On sexual choice in evolutionary thought more broadly, see Erika Lorraine Milam, *Looking for a Few Good Males: Female Choice in Evolutionary Biology* (Baltimore, MD: Johns Hopkins University Press, 2010).
14. Cynthia Eagle Russett describes Darwin's "bitter disappointment at Wallace's defection" in *Sexual Science: The Victorian Construction of Womanhood* (Cambridge, MA: Harvard University Press, 1989), 87.
15. Alfred Russel Wallace, *Contributions to the Theory of Natural Selection: A Series of Essays*, 2nd edition (New York: Macmillan, 1871), 356.

16. Ibid., 359.

17. T. R. R. Stebbing, "Instinct and Reason," *Report and Transactions of the Devonshire Association for the Advancement of Science, Literature, and Art* 4:1 (1870): 155.

18. Ibid., 155–56.

19. Ibid., 155.

20. Darwin, *Descent of Man*, 376, n. 19.

21. Ibid., 360.

22. Ibid., 370.

23. Ibid., 371.

24. Ibid., 384. On this point, see Alys Eve Weinbaum, "Sexual Selection and the Birth of Psychoanalysis: Darwin, Freud, and the Universalization of Wayward Reproduction," in *Wayward Reproductions: Genealogies of Race and Nation in Transatlantic Modern Thought* (Durham, NC: Duke University Press, 2004), 145.

25. Darwin, *Descent of Man*, 377.

26. Ibid., 380.

27. Ibid., 383. Darwin further notes that sexual selection was much more favorable in the (unspecified) "very early period," when man was "guided more by his instinctive passions, and less by foresight or reason" (383).

28. Richard Grant White, *The Fall of Man; or, The Loves of the Gorillas* (New York: Carleton, 1871).

29. White, *The Fall of Man*, 29.

30. Ibid., 29–30.

31. Ibid., 33.

32. Ibid.

33. Ibid., 33–34.

34. Ibid., 34–35.

35. Ibid., 36.

36. Ibid.

37. Ronald L. Numbers, *Darwinism Comes to America* (Cambridge, MA: Harvard University Press, 1998); Paul F. Boller, *American Thought in Transition: The Impact of Evolutionary Naturalism* (Washington, DC: University Press of America, 1981); Milam, *Looking for a Few Good Males*; Kimberly Hamlin, *From Eve to Evolution: Darwin, Science, and Women's Rights in Gilded Age America* (Chicago: University of Chicago Press, 2014).

38. See J. Sokolov, "Julia Pastrana and Her Child," trans. M. Ralston, *The Lancet*, May 3, 1862, 467–69; "Mummies," *Littell's Living Age*, 469–71; "Death of the Bearded Lady," *Saturday Evening Post*, June 9, 1860, 7; Jan

Bondeson, *A Cabinet of Medical Curiosities* (Ithaca, NY: Cornell University Press, 1997), 230–31; Rebecca Stern, "Our Bear Women, Ourselves: Affiliating with Julia Pastrana," in *Victorian Freaks: The Social Context of Freakery in Britain*, ed. Marlene Tromp (Columbus: Ohio State University Press, 2008), 199–233; Rosemarie Garland-Thompson, "Narratives of Deviance and Delight Staring at Julia Pastrana, the 'Extraordinary Lady,'" in *Beyond the Binary: Reconstructing Cultural Identity in a Multicultural Context*, ed. Tim Powell (New Brunswick, NJ: Rutgers University Press, 1990); Kimberly Hamlin, "'The Case of a Bearded Woman': Hypertrichosis and the Construction of Gender in the Age of Darwin," *American Quarterly* 63 (December 2011): 955–981. On pre-Darwinian representations of the spectacularly hairy, see Mary E. Fissell, "Hairy Women and Naked Truths: Gender and the Politics of Knowledge in *Aristotle's Masterpiece*," *William and Mary Quarterly* 60:1 (January 2003): 43–75; Katharine Park and Lorraine J. Daston, "Unnatural Conceptions: The Study of Monsters in Sixteenth- and Seventeenth-Century France and England," *Past and Present* 92 (August 1981): 20–54; Timothy Husband and Gloria Gilmore-House, *The Wild-Man: Medieval Myth and Symbolism* (New York: Metropolitan Museum of Art, 1980), 100–101.

39. Pamphlet, "Account of Miss Pastrana the Nondescript and the Double-Bodied Boy," (London: E. Hancock, c. 1860), Harvard Theatre Collection, Houghton Library, Harvard University; emphasis in original. See also Christopher Hals Gylseth and Lars O. Toverud, *Julia Pastrana: The Tragic Story of the Victorian Ape Woman*, trans. Donald Tumasonis (Stroud, Gloucestershire, England: Sutton, 2003); Linda C. Edsell, *Female Hirsutism: An Enigma: Causes and Treatment of Excess Hair* (St. Louis, MO: Pulsar, 1984); Bondeson, "The Strange Story of Julia Pastrana," in *Cabinet*, 216–44.

40. Charles Darwin, *The Variation of Animals and Plants under Domestication*, vol. 2 (New York: Appleton, 1900 [1868]), 311; *Every Saturday: A Journal of Choice Reading*, July 8, 1871, 31; Bondeson, *Cabinet*, 223.

41. *Every Saturday*, 31.

42. See, e.g., "Farnini's Wonder of Wonders: 'Krao,' a Living Specimen of Darwin's 'Missing Link.'" Postcard pencil dated September 22, 1884, Box 493, "Images—Freaks—Women," Harvard Theatre Collection, Houghton Library, Harvard University; A. H. Keane, "Krao: The 'Human Monkey,'" *Nature*, January 11, 1883, 245–46; Nadja Durbach, "The Missing Link and the Hairy Belle: Krao and the Victorian Discourses of Evolution, Imperialism, and Primitive Sexuality," in *Victorian Freaks: The Social Context of*

Freakery in Britain, ed. Marlene Tromp (Columbus: Ohio State University Press, 2008), 134–53.

43. Frank Crozer Knowles, "Hypertrichiasis in Childhood: The So-Called 'Dog-Faced Boy,'" *Pennsylvania Medical Journal* 24 (March 1921): 403.

44. Janet Browne notes that Darwin alone among Victorian evolutionists was depicted as an ape. See "Darwin in Caricature: A Study in the Popularisation and Dissemination of Evolution," *Proceedings of the American Philosophical Society* 145:4 (December 2001): 507.

45. "Our Hair," *Every Saturday: A Journal of Choice Reading*, May 10, 1873, 520, 521, 523.

46. Darwin, *Variation of Animals*, 307.

47. C. Krebs, "Case of Hypertrichosis (Homo Hirsutus)," trans. H. J. Garrigues, *Archives of Dermatology* 5 (1879 [1878]): 161–62.

48. Henrietta P. Johnson, "Facial Blemishes," in *An International System of Electro-Therapeutics for Students, General Practitioners, and Specialists*, ed. Horatio Bigelow (Philadelphia: Davis, 1894), n.p.

49. Carol Groneman, *Nymphomania* (New York: Norton, 2001); Jean-Charles Sournia, *A History of Alcoholism* (Oxford: Blackwell, 1990).

50. Plymmon S. Hayes, *Electricity and the Method of Its Employment in Removing Superfluous Hair and Other Facial Blemishes* (Chicago: McIntosh Battery and Optical Co., 1894), 24.

51. Ernest L. McEwen, "The Problem of Hypertrichosis," *Journal of Cutaneous Diseases including Syphilis* 35 (1917): 830. See also Knowles, "Hypertrichiasis," 403; Andrew J. Gilmour, "Hypertrichosis," *Journal of Cutaneous Diseases* 36 (April 1918): 255. It is worth emphasizing that many if not most of these physicians perceived "racial" differences between Jews, Celts, Russians, Italians, and Anglo-Saxons. On the history of whiteness in the United States, see Noel Ignatiev, *How the Irish Became White* (New York: Routledge, 1995); Matthew Frye Jacobson, *Whiteness of a Different Color: European Immigrants and the Alchemy of Race* (Cambridge, MA: Harvard University Press, 1999); Karen Brodkin, *How Jews Became White Folks and What That Says about Race in America* (New Brunswick, NJ: Rutgers University Press, 1999); David R. Roediger, *Working toward Whiteness: How America's Immigrants Became White* (New York: Basic Books, 2006).

52. Charles E. Gibbs, "Sexual Behavior and Secondary Sexual Hair in Female Patients with Manic-Depressive Psychoses, and the Relation of These Factors to Dementia Praecox," *American Journal of Psychiatry*, July 4, 1924, 45.

53. Hayes, *Electricity*, 32. See also Gibbs, "Sexual Behavior," 45.

54. Lawrence K. McCafferty, "Hypertrichosis and Its Treatment," *New York Medical Journal,* December 5, 1923, 686.

55. Ibid., 685.

56. Adolph Brand, "Hypertrichosis," *New York Medical Journal,* April 5, 1913, 707.

57. James C. White, "The Use of Electrolysis in the Treatment of Hirsuties," *Boston Medical and Surgical Journal,* May 5, 1881, 412.

58. L. Brocq, "One Hundred and Ten Patients Suffering with Hypertrichosis Treated by Electrolysis," *Annales de Dermatologie et de Syphilologie* 8 (1897), cited in "Selections," *Journal of Cutaneous and Genito-Urinary Diseases* 16 (1898): 200.

59. Johnson, "Facial Blemishes."

60. McEwen, "Problem of Hypertrichosis," 830.

61. Siobhan B. Somerville, "Scientific Racism and the Invention of the Homosexual Body," in *Queering the Color Line: Race and the Invention of Homosexuality in American Culture* (Durham, NC: Duke University Press, 2000), 25.

62. Somerville, "Scientific Racism," 18; George Chauncey, "From Sexual Inversion to Homosexuality: Medicine and the Changing Conceptualization of Female Deviance," in *Passion and Power: Sexuality in History,* ed. Kathy Peiss and Christina Simmons (Philadelphia: Temple University Press, 1989 [1982]), 87–117; Erin G. Carlston, "'A Finer Differentiation': Female Homosexuality and the American Medical Community, 1926–1940," in *Science and Homosexualities,* ed. Vernon A. Rosario (New York: Routledge, 1997), 177–96; Vern L. Bullough, *Science in the Bedroom: A History of Sex Research* (New York: Basic Books, 1994); Chandak Sengoopta, "Glandular Politics: Experimental Biology, Clinical Medicine, and Homosexual Emancipation in Fin-de-Siècle Central Europe," *Isis* 89 (1998): 453.

63. Richard von Krafft-Ebing, *Psychopathia Sexualis: With Especial Reference to the Antipathic Sexual Instinct* (New York: Rebman, 1922 [1886]), 42.

64. Ibid., 43.

65. Ibid., 42. For a thorough analysis of this belief, see Nancy Leys Stepan, "Race and Gender: The Role of Analogy in Science," *Isis* 77 (1986): 261–77.

66. Havelock Ellis, *Studies in the Psychology of Sex: Sexual Inversion* (Philadelphia: Davis, 1901 [1897]), 171. For other references to body hair in the book, see 99, 92, 12, 266, 114, 231, 172.

67. Magnus Hirschfeld, *Die Homosexualität des Mannes und des Weibes,* 2nd edition (Berlin: Marcus, 1920), cited in Sengoopta, "Glandular Politics," 453.

68. See, e.g., von Krafft-Ebing, *Psychopathia Sexualis*, 43, 46.

69. von Krafft-Ebing, *Psychopathia Sexualis*, 332.

70. See, e.g., von Krafft-Ebing, *Psychopathia Sexualis*, 333.

71. Havelock Ellis, "Sexual Inversion in Women," *Alienist and Neurologist* 16:2 (April 1895): 153; Somerville, "Scientific Racism," 18.

72. Ellis, *Studies*, 171.

73. Husband and Gilmore-House, *Wild-Man*, 9–10.

74. Julian Carter, "Normality, Whiteness, Authorship: Evolutionary Sexology and the Primitive Pervert," in *Science and Homosexualities*, ed. Vernon A. Rosario (New York: Routledge, 1997), 155; Somerville, "Scientific Racism," 31.

75. "Medical Jurisprudence: A New Physiological Test of Insanity," *American Law Journal* 11:1 (July 1851): 21–22; "A New Physiological Test for Insanity," *Scientific American*, June 7, 1851.

76. Knowles, "Hypertrichiasis," 403; Daniel H. Tuke, "How the Feelings Affect the Hair," *Popular Science Monthly*, December 1872, 158–61; idem, "Illustrations of the Influence of the Mind upon the Body in Health and Disease," *Journal of Mental Science* 18 (April 1872): 8–31. On Virchow, see Nigel Rothfels, *Savages and Beasts: The Birth of the Modern Zoo* (Baltimore. MD: Johns Hopkins University Press, 2002), 99–100; Bruce Lincoln, *Theorizing Myth: Narrative, Ideology, and Scholarship* (Chicago: University of Chicago Press, 1999), 105–6, 252 n. 15.

77. Benjamin Godfrey, *Diseases of Hair: A Popular Treatise upon the Affections of the Hair System* (Philadelphia: Lindsay and Blakiston, 1872), 31.

78. "Diseases of the Hair [Hypertrichiasis and Mental Derangement]," *Annual of the Universal Medical Sciences*, ed. Charles E. Sajous, vol. 4 (Philadelphia: Davis, 1893), A-28.

79. Havelock Ellis, *The Criminal*, 5th edition (New York: Scribner's, 1900[?]), 79–80. Ellis here echoes Cesare Lombroso and William Ferrero's conclusions in *The Female Offender*, ed. W. Douglas Morrison (London: Fisher, 1895).

80. See, for example, Fissell, "Hairy Women," 43–75; Joan Cadden, *Meanings of Sexual Difference in the Middle Ages: Medicine, Science, and Culture* (Cambridge: Cambridge University Press, 1993), 203–4; Husband and Gilmore-House, *The Wild-Man*, 100–101.

81. Bernarr Macfadden, *Hair Culture: Rational Methods for Growing the Hair and for Developing Its Strength and Beauty* (Bedford, MA: Applewood, 2000 [1922]), 158. See also Sharra L. Vostral, *Under Wraps: A History of Menstrual Hygiene Technology* (Lanham, MD: Lexington, 2008), chap. 3; Carroll Smith-Rosenberg, *Disorderly Conduct: Visions of Gender in Victorian Amer-*

ica (New York: Oxford University Press, 1986); Russett, *Sexual Science*; G. J. Barker-Benfield, *The Horrors of the Half-Known Life: Male Attitudes toward Women and Sexuality in 19th Century America* (New York: Routledge, 1999).

82. George Henry Fox, "On the Permanent Removal of Hair by Electrolysis," *Medical Record* 15 (1879): 270.

NOTES TO CHAPTER 4

1. Paul E. Bechet, "The Etiology and Treatment of Hypertrichosis," *New York Medical Journal*, August 16, 1913, 313.

2. H. C. Baum, "The Etiology and Treatment of Superfluous Hair," *Journal of the American Medical Association* 54 (1912): 104.

3. Herman Goodman, "The Problem of Excess Hair," *Hygeia* 8 (May 1930): 433; Maurice Costello, "How to Remove Superfluous Hair," *Hygeia* 18 (July 1940): 586; William J. Young, "Hypertrichosis and Its Treatment," *Kentucky Medical Journal* 18 (June 1920): 217; Oscar L. Levin, "Superfluous Hair," *Good Housekeeping*, September 1928, 106. While empathetic physicians and beauty specialists focused on the intense suffering endured by hairy women, the presence of body hair did not necessarily lead women to melancholia or suicide. At least a few women viewed their bountiful body hair as neither "excessive" nor merely adequate but instead as a beautiful complement to the rest of their physiques. See, e.g., Joseph Mitchell, "Profiles: Lady Olga," *New Yorker*, August 3, 1940, 20–28.

4. Mrs. H. J. Leek to *Journal of the AMA*, 19 February 19, 1937, folder 0318-06, American Medical Association Historical Health Fraud Collection, Chicago (hereafter cited as AMA).

5. Miss J. Mamolite to AMA, February 17, 1943, folder 0318-06, AMA.

6. Mrs. A. T. Hutto to *Hygeia*, January 15, 1932, folder 0317-16, AMA. See also Marie Fink to AMA, August 17, 1931, folder 0317-02, AMA; Mrs. B. Tellef to AMA, August 6, 1926, folder 0318-01, AMA; Mrs. Allen Stamper to *Hygeia*, November 4, 1929, folder 0317-03, AMA.

7. See Laura L. Behling, *The Masculine Woman in America, 1890–1935* (Urbana: University of Illinois Press, 2001); Martha Vicinus, "'They Wonder to Which Sex I Belong': The Historical Roots of Modern Lesbian Identity," in *The Lesbian and Gay Studies Reader*, ed. Henry Abelone, Michéle Aina Barale, and David M. Halperin (New York: Routledge, 1993), 432–52; Carroll Smith-Rosenberg, *Disorderly Conduct: Visions of Gender in Victorian America* (New York: Oxford University Press, 1985); Rosalyn Terborg-Penn, "African American Women and the Woman Suffrage Movement,"

in *One Woman, One Vote: Rediscovering the Woman Suffrage Movement*, ed. Marjorie Spruill Wheeler (Troutdale, OR: New Sage, 1995), 135–55.

8. Herbert J. Claiborne, "Hypertrichosis in Women: Its Relation to Bisexuality (Hermaphroditism): With Remarks on Bisexuality in Animals, Especially Man," *New York Medical Journal*, June 13, 1914, 1183.

9. John D'Emilio and Estelle B. Freedman, *Intimate Matters: A History of Sexuality in America* (New York: Harper & Row, 1988), 222–35; Christina Simmons, "African Americans and Sexual Victorianism in the Social Hygiene Movement, 1910–1940," *Journal of the History of Sexuality* 4:1 (July 1993): 51–75; Elizabeth Lunbeck, "'A New Generation of Women': Progressive Psychiatrists and the Hypersexual Female," *Feminist Studies* 13 (1987): 535–36; George Chauncey, "From Sexual Inversion to Homosexuality: Medicine and the Changing Conceptualization of Female Deviance," in *Passion and Power: Sexuality in History*, ed. Kathy Peiss and Christina Simmons (Philadelphia: Temple University Press, 1989), 87–117.

10. Vincent Vinikas, *Soft Soap, Hard Sell: American Hygiene in an Age of Advertisement* (Ames: Iowa State University Press, 1992), 45–77; Eve Weinbaum, Priti Ramamurthy, Lynn M. Thomas, Uta G. Poiger, Madeline Yue Dong, and Tani E. Barlow, *The Modern Girl around the World: Consumption, Modernity, and Globalization* (Durham, NC: Duke University Press, 2009).

11. On "in-betweenness," see David R. Roediger, *Working toward Whiteness: How America's Immigrants Became White* (New York: Basic Books, 2006), chapter 3. Also see T. J. Jackson Lears, "American Advertising and the Reconstruction of the Body, 1880–1930," in *Fitness in American Culture: Images of Health, Sport, and the Body, 1830–1940*, ed. Kathryn Grover (Amherst: University of Massachusetts Press, 1989), 56; Nancy Tomes, *The Gospel of Germs: Men, Women, and the Microbe in American Life* (Cambridge, MA: Harvard University Press, 1998); Lara Friedenfelds, *The Modern Period: Menstruation in Twentieth-Century America* (Baltimore, MD: Johns Hopkins University Press, 2009); Vinikas, *Soft Soap, Hard Sell*, 79–117.

12. Joan Jacobs Brumberg, *The Body Project: An Intimate History of American Girls* (New York: Random House, 1997), 98; Doreen Yarwood, *Fashion in the Western World, 1500–1990* (London: Batsford, 1992); Valerie Mendes and Amy De La Haye, *20th-Century Fashion* (London: Thames & Hudson, 1999); Jacqueline Herald, *Fashions of a Decade: The 1920s* (New York: Facts on File, 1991); Kirsten Hansen, "Hair or Bare? The History of American Women and Hair Removal, 1914–1934," Senior Thesis in American Studies, Barnard College (April 2007); Christine Hope, "Caucasian Female Body

Hair and American Culture," *Journal of American Culture* 5 (Spring 1982): 93–99.

13. Edward Bok, cited in Lisa Belicka Keränen, "'Girls Who Come to Pieces': Women, Cosmetics, and Advertising in the *Ladies' Home Journal*, 1900–1920," in *Turning the Century: Essays in Media and Cultural Studies*, ed. Carol A. Stabile (Boulder, CO: Westview Press, 2000), 147. Also see Erin G. Carlston, "'A Finer Differentiation': Female Homosexuality and the American Medical Community, 1926–1940," in *Science and Homosexualities*, ed. Vernon A. Rosario (New York: Routledge, 1997), 178; Vinikas, *Soft Soap, Hard Sell*. Although the history of clothing tends to be studied as indicative of "deeper" socioeconomic transformations, Valerie Steele has argued that "the evolution of fashion has an internal dynamic of its own that is only very gradually and tangentially affected by social change within the wider culture" (*Fashion and Eroticism: Ideals of Feminine Beauty from the Victorian Era to the Jazz Age* [New York: Oxford University Press, 1985], 5). Whether explained by "internal" or external factors, shifts in Americans' prevailing modes of dress certainly altered concern with body hair.

14. T. S. Eliot, "The Love Song of J. Alfred Prufrock," *Complete Poems and Plays, 1909–1950* (New York: Harcourt, Brace, 1952). For further discussion see William Ian Miller, *The Anatomy of Disgust* (Cambridge, MA: Harvard University Press, 1997), 56.

15. Kathleen Endres and Therese Lueck, eds., *Women's Periodicals in the United States: Consumer Magazines* (Westport, CT: Greenwood, 1995); Bonnie Fox, "Selling the Mechanized Household: 70 Years of Ads in *Ladies Home Journal*," *Gender and Society* 4 (1990): 25–40.

16. Hope, "Caucasian Female Body Hair," 94; G. Bruce Retallack, "Razors, Shaving, and Gender Construction: An Inquiry into the Material Culture of Shaving," *Material History Review* 49 (Spring 1999): 8; Ellen van Oost, "Materialized Gender: How Shavers Configure the Users' Femininity and Masculinity," in *How Users Matter: The Co-Construction of Users and Technologies*, ed. Nelly Oudshoorn and Trevor Pinch (Cambridge, MA: MIT Press, 2003), 200. Searches in the Readex database of African American and Hispanic American newspapers indicate no similar increase in hair removal advertisements.

17. *McClure's Magazine*, March/April 1920, 90; *McClure's Magazine*, May 1920, 60; *McClure's Magazine*, June 1920, 2.

18. Flyer stamped October 2, 1912, AMA Folder 0315-08.

19. See, e.g., Delmar Emil Bordeaux, *Cosmetic Electrolysis and the Removal of Superfluous Hair* (Rockford, IL: Bellevue, 1942); Anna Hazelton Delavan,

"Superfluous Hair," *Good Housekeeping*, March 1925, 96; Joseph Rohrer, *Rohrer's Illustrated Book on Scientific Modern Beauty Culture* (New York: Rohrer's Institute of Beauty Culture, 1924), 46.

20. This choreography of constraint and freedom also appeared in emerging norms of thinness. See Peter N. Stearns, *Fat History: Bodies and Beauty in the Modern West* (New York: New York University Press, 1997), 54.

21. Peter N. Stearns, *Battleground of Desire: The Struggle for Self-Control in Modern America* (New York: New York University Press, 1999), 99–100; Hope, "Caucasian Female Body Hair," 93–99; Susan Brownmiller, *Femininity* (New York: Simon & Schuster, 1984), 142–48; Christy Callahan, "Body Hair Removal in the United States from a Social Historical Perspective," *Oakland Review* 23 (1996): 74–83; Lears, "American Advertising," 47–66.

22. Knight Dunlap, *Personal Beauty and Racial Betterment* (St. Louis, MO: Mosby, 1920), 40.

23. Alfred F. Niemoeller, *Superfluous Hair and Its Removal* (New York: Harvest House, 1938), 13.

24. Advertisement for the Velvet Mitten Company, Los Angeles, folder 0317-01, AMA; Geyser, "Truth and Fallacy concerning the Roentgen Ray in Hypertrichosis," *Scientific Therapy and Practical Research* (March 1926), reprint in folder 0317-17, AMA.

25. Geyser, "Truth and Fallacy."

26. M. C. Phillips, *Skin Deep: The Truth about Beauty Aids—Safe and Harmful* (New York: Vanguard, 1934), 91. For more recent reports of severe ulcerations caused by calcium thioglycolate depilatories, see Alexander A. Fisher, "Unique Reactions of Scrotal Skin to Topical Agents," *Cutis* 44 (December 1989): 445.

27. Miss M.C. to *Chicago Tribune* (undated, circa November 1915), AMA Folder 0315-08.

28. On Koremlu, see *Journal of the American Medical Association*, July 30, 1932, 407; A. J. Cramp, *Nostrums and Quackery and Pseudo-Medicine*, vol. 3 (Chicago, 1936), 35; and Gwen Kay, *Dying to Be Beautiful: The Fight for Safe Cosmetics* (Columbus: Ohio State University Press, 2005). One writer noted in 1931 that Koremlu is "widely advertised, and in all the better class magazines." Moreover, "from inquiries made at various department stores in surrounding cities it is undoubtedly being used, and I was assured that there had been no complaint on it, nothing but praise, in fact. . . . [O]ne store stated that a local physician had been purchasing it." See N. H. Franz to AMA, December 19, 1931, folder 0316-06, AMA.

29. Cited in Niemoeller, *Superfluous Hair*, 48.

30. Young, "Hypertrichosis," 217; Niemoeller, *Superfluous Hair*, 91; Trotter, "Hair Growth and Shaving," *Anatomical Record* 37 (1928): 373–79.

31. Ernst Ludwig Franz Kroymayer, *The Cosmetic Treatment of Skin Complaints* (London: Oxford University Press, 1930), 69; Ernest L. McEwen, "The Problem of Hypertrichosis," *Journal of Cutaneous Diseases including Syphilis* 35 (1917): 832.

32. Rebecca Herzig, "Subjected to the Current: Batteries, Bodies, and the Early History of Electrification in the United States," *Journal of Social History* (Summer 2008): 867–85.

33. As technical refinements were made to electrolysis equipment, the procedure was also practiced at home. See Niemoeller, *Superfluous Hair*, chap. 21.

34. Adolph Brand, "Hypertrichosis," *New York Medical Journal* 97 (1913): 708. Also see S. Sorenson, "Practical Removal of Hairs, Moles, etc., by Electrolysis," *Medical News*, September 30, 1893, 371.

35. L. Brocq, "One Hundred and Ten Patients Suffering with Hypertrichosis Treated by Electrolysis," *Annales de Dermatologie et de Syphilologie* 8 (1897), cited in "Selections," *Journal of Cutaneous and Genito-Urinary Diseases* 16 (1898): 198.

36. Brand, "Hypertrichosis," 708; Young, "Hypertrichosis," 218–19.

37. While historians typically resist explaining technological diffusion according to "utility" (the idea that certain technologies succeed simply because they work better than others), the efficacy of x-ray hair removal was widely acknowledged in the early twentieth century. See AMA to Mrs. P. G. Range, October 28, 1927, folder 0314-03, AMA; AMA to Mr. A. E. Backman, May 29, 1930, folder 0314-03, AMA.

38. Mary Mulholland to AMA, May 20, 1930, folder 0318-02, AMA. This description of the Tricho Machine may remind some readers of the shoe-fitting fluoroscopes employed in North American and European shoe stores in the mid-twentieth century. See "Shoe-Fitting Fluoroscopes," *Journal of the American Medical Association*, April 9, 1949, 1004-5; H. Kopp, "Radiation Damage Caused by Shoe-Fitting Fluoroscope," *British Medical Journal* 2 (1957): 1344-45; Jacalyn Duffin and Charles R. R. Hayter, "Baring the Sole: The Rise and Fall of the Shoe-Fitting Fluroscope," *Isis* 91 (2000): 260–82.

39. Geyser, "Facts and Fallacies about the Removal of Superfluous Hair," folder 0317-17, AMA.

40. Mary P. Searles to AMA, October 16, 1925, folder 0318-01, AMA.

41. Nellie M. Moore to AMA, October 10, 1951, folder 0317-12, AMA.

42. Mrs. Jennie Stedman Farrell to AMA, September 25, 1925, folder 0318-01, AMA; C. A. Harper, M.D., to A. J. Cramp, June 10, 1927, folder 0318-01, AMA.

43. Mrs. Jennie Stedman Farrell to AMA, September 25, 1925, folder 0318-01, AMA.

44. See, for example, Lucille M. Naess to AMA, November 14, 1949, folder 0314-05, AMA, and the reply from the AMA (November 18, 1949).

45. For example, twelve former x-ray clients studied by two Canadian physicians in 1989 reported that the specialist who operated their x-ray salon was herself a former x-ray recipient undergoing treatment for cancer. The former clients described this specialist as a "mother-like nurse," and none of the twelve would provide the investigating physicians with the operator's name for fear that the woman might be subject to prosecution. See Irving B. Rosen and Paul G. Walfish, "Sequelae of Radiation Facial Epilation (North American Hiroshima Maiden Syndrome)," *Surgery* 106 (December 1989): 947. Also see "Memo to Mr. Cantor concerning Visit to Keat, Inc.," December 4, 1947, file marked "Superfluous Hair Removal (Keat)," collection of Mr. Bob McCoy, Museum of Questionable Medical Devices, Minneapolis, Minnesota.

46. "Gone for Good," advertisement for Rudolph Tricho Institute, Detroit, folder 0318-01, AMA.

47. E.g., "Tricho Method of Removing Superfluous Hair," advertisement for Mrs. L. P. Williams's Tricho salons, Connecticut and Massachusetts, folder 0318-01, AMA.

48. "Loveliness for the Most Discriminating Women," advertisement for Hair-X Salon, Philadelphia, folder 0317-02, AMA.

49. "A Flawless Skin," *Boston Post*, November 15, 1928, copy in folder 0318-02, AMA.

50. "Gone for Good."

51. Lois Banner, *American Beauty* (Chicago: University of Chicago Press, 1983), 205.

52. On the immediate public response to Roentgen's announcement, see Nancy Knight, "The New Light: X-Rays and Medical Futurism," in *Imagining Tomorrow: History, Technology, and the American Future*, ed. Joseph J. Corn (Cambridge, MA: MIT Press, 1986); Ronald L. Eisenberg, *Radiology: An Illustrated History* (St. Louis: Mosby-Year Book, 1992); E. R. N. Grigg, *The Trail of the Invisible Light* (Springfield, IL: Thomas, 1965); Ruth Brecher and Edward Brecher, *The Rays: A History of Radiology in the United States and Canada* (Baltimore, MD: Williams and Wilkins, 1969).

53. John Daniel, "The X-rays," *Science*, April 10, 1896, 562–63.

54. Brecher and Brecher, *Rays*, 81, 82.

55. Eduard Schiff and Leopold Freund, "Beiträge zur Radiotherapie," *Weiner*

Medicinische Wochenschrift, May 28, 1898, 1058–61.

56. Neville Wood, "Depilation by Roentgen Rays," *Lancet*, January 27, 1900, 231; T. Sjögren and E. Sederholm, "Beitrag zur therapeutischen Verwertung der Röntgenstrahlen," *Fortschritte auf dem Gebiete der Röntgenstrahlen* 4 (1901): 145–70; Edith R. Meek, "A Variety of Skin Lesions Treated by X-ray," *Boston Medical and Surgical Journal*, August 7, 1902, 152–53.

57. Mihran Krikor Kassabian, *Röntgen Rays and Electro-therapeutics* (Philadelphia: Lippincott, 1910), 80.

58. V. E. A. Pullin and W. J. Wiltshire, *X-Rays Past and Present* (London, 1927), 173–74.

59. Brecher and Brecher, *Rays*, chap. 7.

60. On "martyrs" to the x-ray, see Rebecca M. Herzig, *Suffering for Science: Reason and Sacrifice in Modern America* (New Brunswick, NJ: Rutgers University Press, 2005), chap. 5.

61. Paul Starr, *The Social Transformation of American Medicine* (New York: Basic Books, 1982); Joel Howell, *Technology in the Hospital* (Baltimore, MD: Johns Hopkins University Press, 1995); Stanley Joel Reiser, *Medicine and the Reign of Technology* (New York: Cambridge University Press, 1978); Bettyann Holtzmann Kevles, *Naked to the Bone: Medical Imaging in the Twentieth Century* (New Brunswick, NJ: Rutgers University Press, 1997); Lisa Cartwright, *Screening the Body: Tracing Medicine's Visual Culture* (Minneapolis: University of Minnesota Press, 1995), esp. chap. 5.

62. George M. MacKee, "Hypertrichosis and the X-ray," *Journal of Cutaneous Diseases including Syphilis* 35 (1917): 177.

63. Carl Beck, *Röntgen Ray Diagnosis and Therapy* (New York, 1904), 377.

64. William Allen Pusey and Eugene Wilson Caldwell, *Röntgen Rays in Therapeutics and Diagnosis* (Philadelphia, 1904), 360–61. On professionalizing physicians' exclusion of cosmetic practices and practitioners during the first two decades of the twentieth century, see Beth Haiken, "Plastic Surgery and American Beauty at 1921," *Bulletin of the History of Medicine* 68 (1994): 429–53.

65. Although most professional physicians had disavowed x-ray hair removal by 1918, it is important to note that this rejection was neither uniform nor total. As late as 1927 two physicians in Chicago offered an epilating dose of x-rays to a girl with a hairy chin and upper lip (Mrs. P. G. Range to A. J. Cramp, 23 October 1927, folder 0314-03, AMA); three years later, physician H. H. Hazen reported other colleagues still practicing x-ray hair removal (H. H. Hazen, "Injuries Resulting in Irradiation in Beauty Shops," *American Journal of Roentgenology and Radium Therapy* 23 [1930]: 411). Some

evidence hints at the medical use of x-ray hair removal as late as 1960. See Howard T. Behrman, "Diagnosis and Management of Hirsutism," *Journal of the American Medical Association*, April 23, 1960, 126.

66. See, e.g., "With the Advancement of Science Comes the Modern Way to Remove Superfluous Hair Permanently: TRICHO SYSTEM," advertisement for Tricho salon, Boston, folder 0317-17, AMA.

67. "Permanent Freedom from Unwanted Hair," advertisement for the Virginia Laboratories, AMA folder 0317-01. Baltimore's Virginia Laboratories employed the "Marton Method," and used Marton's text and illustrations in many of their advertisements.

68. On the "strange powers" of the ray, see "Gone for Good."

69. Ibid.

70. "Be Your True Self: We Will Tell You How," advertisement for Frances A. Post, Inc., Cleveland, folder 0317-01, AMA.

71. "Beauty Is Your Heritage," advertisement for Marveau Laboratories, Chicago, folder 0317-02, AMA; "With the Advancement of Science"; Albert C. Geyser, M.D., "Facts and Fallacies about the Removal of Superfluous Hair," folder 0317-17, AMA; "Loveliness for the Most Discriminating Women," advertisement for Hair-X Salon, Philadelphia, folder 0317-02, AMA.

72. H. Gellert [Secretary of Hamomar Institute] to "Madam," 1933, folder 0317-01, AMA.

73. Copy of letter, Miss H. Stearn to National Institute of Health, July 5, 1933, folder 0317-01, AMA; "BEAUTY: Woman's Most Precious Gift" [advertisement for the Dermic Laboratories, San Francisco and Los Angeles], folder 0317-02, AMA.

74. M. J. Rush, "Hypertrichosis: The Marton Method, a Triumph of Chemistry," *Medical Practice*, March 1924, 956, reprint in folder 0317-01, AMA.

75. "Beauty Is Your Heritage."

76. "Permanent Freedom from Unwanted Hair," folder 0317-02, AMA.

77. Herman Goodman, "Correspondence," *Journal of the American Medical Association*, May 9, 1925, 1443; S. Dana Hubbard [City of New York Department of Public Health] to A. J. Cramp, January 8, 1929, folder 0318-02, AMA; Dale Brown [Cleveland Better Business Bureau] to A. J. Cramp, July 29, 1930, folder 0314-03; AMA. Even if x-ray salons recorded statistics on their clients' racial and ethnic backgrounds, these classifications would not necessarily coincide with clients' self-identifications, nor with twenty-first-century racial and ethnic typologies.

78. Some men expressed concern that adopting this method of hair removal— a method marketed so strongly to women—might cause them to become

"effeminate." See, e.g., Arthur Nelson to AMA, ca. July 20, 1934, folder 0317-01, AMA.

79. Edward Oliver, "Dermatitis Due to 'Tricho Method,'" *Archives of Dermatology and Syphilology* 25 (1932): 948; D. E. Cleveland, "The Removal of Superfluous Hair by X-Rays," *Canadian Medical Association Journal* 59 (1948): 375.

80. Internal Memo from B. O. Halling, October 22, 1925, folder 0318-01, AMA; Mary Mulholland to AMA, May 20, 1930, AMA, folder 0318-02; Mrs. B. Tellef to AMA, August 6, 1926, folder 0318-01, AMA. Many women received more than forty treatments; one young woman received *fourteen hundred* exposures over five years. See the case reported by Dorothy R. Kirk to Arthur Cramp, December 14, 1928, folder 0315-14, AMA.

81. One 1947 investigation concluded that thousands of Americans visited a single x-ray hair removal company alone, the Tricho Sales Corporation (A. C. Cipollaro and M. B. Einhorn, "Use of X-Rays for Treatment of Hypertrichosis Is Dangerous," *Journal of the American Medical Association*, October 11, 1947, 350). Tricho advertisements boasted that their method of hair removal had been used "by thousands of women long before the discovery was announced to the public," lending further indeterminacy to the number of individuals using x-ray hair removal (e.g., "The Tricho System," advertisement for George Hoppman's salon, Chicago, folder 0318-01, AMA). Since Tricho was just one of dozens of similar x-ray companies in operation, one can conclude that tens of thousands of other Americans also used the technique. On the popularity of x-ray hair removal, also see Lewis Herber [Murray Bookchin], *Our Synthetic Environment* (New York: Knopf, 1962), 166–67.

82. Donna Haraway, "Teddy Bear Patriarchy: Taxidermy in the Garden of Eden, New York City, 1908–1936," in *Primate Visions: Gender, Race, and Nature in the World of Modern Science* (New York, 1989), 26–58.

83. Mary F. Amerise to AMA, May 18, 1925, folder 0314-03, AMA.

84. Anne Steiman to AMA, September 5, 1933, folder 0317-01, AMA.

85. "A Flawless Skin," *Boston Post*, November 15, 1928, copy in folder 0318-02, AMA.

86. Katherine Moore to AMA, August 27, 1931, folder 0318-02, AMA.

87. Copy of memorandum, J. W. Williams to C. B. Pinkham, M.D., March 2, 1940, folder 0317-01, AMA.

88. Ibid.

89. See Levin, "Superfluous Hair," 190–91. On clients' resistance to authorities' condemnations, see H. L. J. Marshall to AMA, May 30, 1928, folder 0318-02, AMA. It should be noted that some women sought medical advice on the

x-ray treatments of superfluous hair, and upon hearing condemnation of the practice, unhesitatingly rejected it. Others, already well informed on the potential dangers of x-ray overexposure, were blatantly misinformed about the nature of the technology by x-ray providers themselves. See, e.g., the report of case from G. V. Stryker, M.D., in "The Tricho System Again," *Journal of the American Medical Association*, March 16, 1929, 919; Mary Mulholland to AMA, June 24, 1930, folder 0318-02, AMA.

90. See Robert Proctor's discussion of changes in postwar eugenic discourse in *Racial Hygiene: Medicine under the Nazis* (Cambridge, MA: Harvard University Press, 1989), 303–8.

91. Anja Hiddinga, "X-ray Technology in Obstetrics: Measuring Pelves at the Yale School of Medicine," in *Medical Innovations in Historical Perspective*, ed. John Pickstone (New York: St. Martin's, 1992), 143; M. Susan Lindee, *Suffering Made Real: American Science and the Survivors at Hiroshima* (Chicago: University of Chicago Press, 1994); Daniel Paul Serwer, "The Rise of Radiation Protection: Science, Medicine, and Technology in Society, 1896–1935," Ph.D. diss., Princeton University, 1976; and Gilbert F. Whittemore, "The National Committee on Radiation Protection, 1928–1960: From Professional Guidelines to Government Regulation," Ph.D. diss., Harvard University, 1986.

92. See N. H. Franz to AMA, December 19, 1931, folder 0316-06, AMA.

93. On the revision of licensing laws, see copy of C. B. Pinkham, M.D., to Max C. Starkhoff, April 3, 1928, folder 0318-02, AMA; C. B. Pinkham to A. J. Cramp, January 22, 1929, folder 0318-02, AMA. On the distribution of x-ray equipment, see A. J. Cramp to Dr. Howard Fox, November 15, 1929, folder 0318-02, AMA; Rollins H. Stevens to Dr. Arthur Cramp, November 8, 1929, folder 0318-02, AMA.

94. Better Business Bureau of Rochester to A. J. Cramp, May 15, 1930, folder 0318-02, AMA; Howard Fox to Dr. Arthur J. Cramp, November 13, 1929, folder 0318-02, AMA; Catherine Caufield, *Multiple Exposures: Chronicles of the Radiation Age* (New York: Harper & Row, 1989).

95. The disintegration of the Tricho Sales Corporation in 1930, for example, was influenced by a collective lawsuit organized by a group of seven New York women, all former clients. See the letter from S. Dana Hubbard, M.D., of the New York City Department of Health to A. J. Cramp, January 8, 1929, folder 0318-02, AMA. See also S. Dana Hubbard to Dr. C. B. Pinkham, January 8, 1929, folder 0318-02, AMA.

96. See, e.g., the case of "Mrs. E.B.," aged thirty, in F. J. Eichenlaub, "Some More Tricho Cases," *Journal of the American Medical Association*, April 26,

1930, 1341. On injuries, also see Cipollaro and Einhorn, "Use of X-Rays," 350; H. Martin et al., "Radiation-Induced Skin Cancer of the Head and Neck," *Cancer* 25 (1970): 61–71; R. A. Schwartz, G. H. Burgess, and H. Milgrom, "Breast Carcinoma and Basal Cell Epithelioma after X-Ray Therapy for Hirsutism," *Cancer* 44:5 (November 1979): 1601–5; Rosen and Walfish, "Sequelae of Radiation Facial Epilation," *Surgery* 106 (December 1989): 946–50.

97. New franchises that publicly advertised the technique were opening in Canada as late as 1948. See Cleveland, "Removal of Superfluous Hair," 374. It is impossible to determine the extent of informal or "back-alley" x-ray hair removal.

98. Helen L. Camp to AMA, March 30, 1954, folder 0318-02, AMA.

NOTES TO CHAPTER 5

1. "Bearded Lady's Gland Cures Addison's Disease," *Science News Letter*, November 16, 1946, 318. The story is particularly alarming given the same publication's claim, sixteen years earlier, that adrenal glands are the most important organ in the body: "Life does not long continue in a body from which they have been removed." See Jane Stafford, "Adrenal Glands Save Our Lives," *Science News-Letter*, March 1, 1930, 132.

2. Stephanie H. Kenen, "Who Counts When You're Counting Homosexuals? Hormones and Homosexuality in Mid-Twentieth-Century America," in *Science and Homosexualities*, ed. Vernon A. Rosario (New York: Routledge, 1997), 201. Also see Joanne Meyerowitz, *How Sex Changed: A History of Transsexuality in the United States* (Cambridge, MA: Harvard University Press, 2002); Nelly Oudshoorn, "Endocrinologists and the Conceptualization of Sex, 1920–1940," *Journal of the History of Biology* 23:2 (Summer 1990): 163–86.

3. German Shapiro and Shmuel Evron, "A Novel Use of Spironolactone: Treatment of Hirsutism," *Journal of Clinical Endocrinology and Metabolism* 51:3 (1980): 429.

4. It is worth remembering that some older depilatories, such as those made from thallium, also worked systemically; but they were so toxic in their effects that they cannot be considered entirely effective drugs. On thallium, see Eugene J. Segre, *Androgens, Virilization, and the Hirsute Female* (Springfield, IL: Thomas, 1967), 88.

5. Aristotle, *History of Animals: In Ten Books* (Whitefish, MT: Kessinger, 2004), 290. See also George Washington Corner, "The Early History of the

Oestrogenic Hormones," *Journal of Endocrinology* 31 (January 1965): iii, xv–xvi; Lu Gwei-Djen and Joseph Needham, "Medieval Preparations of Urinary Steroid Hormones," *Nature*, December 14, 1963, 1047–48.

6. Georges Canguilhem, *The Vital Rationalist: Selected Writings from Georges Canguilhem*, trans. François Delaporte (New York: Zone, 1994), 85; Merriley Borell, "Organotherapy and the Emergence of Reproductive Endocrinology," *Journal of the History of Biology* 18:1 (Spring 1985): 10.

7. Corner, "Early History," iv; Ann Dalley, *Women under the Knife: A History of Surgery* (New York: Routledge, 1991), 146–56; Regina Morantz-Sanchez, "The Making of a Woman Surgeon: How Mary Dixon Jones Made a Name for Herself in Nineteenth-Century Gynecology," in *Women Healers and Physicians: Climbing a Long Hill*, ed. Lillian R. Furst (Lexington: University Press of Kentucky, 1997), 183–84; Richard Harrison Shyrock, *Medicine and Society in America, 1660–1860* (New York: New York University Press, 1960).

8. D. Schultheiss, J. Denil, and U. Jonas, "Rejuvenation in the Early 20th Century," *Andrologia* 29:6 (November–Decemer 1997): 351–55; Corner, "Early History," v; Charles-Edouard Brown-Séquard, "Du role physiologique et thérapeutique d'un suc extrait de testicules d'animaux d'après nombre de faits observes chez l'homme," *Archives de physiologie normale et pathologique* 1 (1889): 739–46.

9. Borell, "Organotherapy," 6; Corner, "Early History," v; Brown-Séquard, "Du role physiologique," 739–46.

10. Edgar Allen and Edward Doisy, "An Ovarian Hormone: Preliminary Report on Its Localization, Extraction, and Partial Purification, and Action in Test Animals," *Journal of the American Medical Association*, September 8, 1923, 820; Borell, "Organotherapy," 3; Merriley Borell, "Brown-Séquard's Organotherapy and Its Appearance in America at the End of the Nineteenth Century," *Bulletin of the History of Medicine* 50 (1976): 312; "Spermine," *Medical and Surgical Reporter*, April 25, 1891, 473–74; Corner, "Early History," x.

11. John P. Swann, *Academic Scientists and the Pharmaceutical Industry: Cooperative Research in Twentieth-Century America* (Baltimore, MD: Johns Hopkins University Press, 1988), 35; Paul Starr, *The Social Transformation of American Medicine* (New York: Basic Books, 1982), 127–34.

12. Corner, "Early History," v.

13. The disrepute of the field stemmed not only from the glands' association with sexual anatomy but also from the lucrative nature of transplanting animal glands into people. Matters could not have been helped by the fact that the work was so technically complicated that many experimenters la-

bored to obtain any measurable effects from the extracts at all. See Celia Roberts, *Messengers of Sex: Hormones, Biomedicine, and Feminism* (New York: Cambridge University Press, 2007), 34 n. 5; Laura Davidow Hirshbein, "The Glandular Solution: Sex, Masculinity, and Aging in the 1920s," *Journal of the History of Sexuality* 9:3 (2000): 277–304; John M. Hoberman and Charles E. Yesalis, "The History of Synthetic Testosterone," *Scientific American*, February 1995, 60–65; Borell, "Organotherapy," 2, 3; Borell, "Brown-Séquard," 309–20; George R. Murray, "Note on the Treatment of Myxoedema by Hypodermic Injections of an Extract of the Thyroid Gland of a Sheep," *British Medical Journal* 2 (1891): 796–97.

14. See, e.g., the advertisements in the *Congregationalist* [Boston], February 14, 1895, 261; the *New York Evangelist*, May 23, 1895, 34; the *Independent* [New York], June 27, 1895, 31; *Watchman* [Boston], July 25, 1895, 23; *Zion's Herald* [Boston], December 4, 1895, 799.

15. Corner, "Early History," vi.

16. Oudshoorn, "Endocrinologists," 168. On raw materials, see Adele E. Clarke, "Research Materials and Reproductive Science in the United States, 1910–1940," in *Physiology in the American Context, 1850–1940*, ed. Gerald L. Geison (Baltimore, MD: American Physiological Society, 1987), 331; Corner, "Early History," xiii.

17. Robert T. Frank, *The Female Sex Hormone* (Springfield, IL: Thomas, 1929), cited in Oudshoorn, "Endocrinologists," 167–68.

18. Corner, "Early History," x; Borell, "Organotherapy," 18.

19. F. G. Young, "The Evolution of Ideas about Animal Hormones," in *The Chemistry of Life: Eight Lectures on the History of Biochemistry*, ed. Joseph Needham (Cambridge: Cambridge University Press, 1970), 126; Diana Long Hall, "The Critic and the Advocate: Contrasting British Views on the State of Endocrinology in the early 1920s," *Journal of the History of Biology* 9:2 (Autumn 1976): 279.

20. Nelly Oudshoorn, *Beyond the Natural Body: An Archaeology of Sex Hormones* (New York: Routledge, 1994), 29; Meyerowitz, *How Sex Changed*, 27–28.

21. Roberts, *Messengers*, 37; Oudshoorn, "Endocrinologists," 164, n. 3.

22. Bernhard Zondek, "Mass Excretion of Oestrogenic Hormone in the Urine of the Stallion," *Nature*, March 31, 1934, 209–10.

23. A. S. Parkes, "The Rise of Reproductive Endocrinology, 1926–1940," *Journal of Endocrinology* 34 (1966): 26.

24. Oudshoorn, "Endocrinologists," 174; Herbert Evans, cited in Diana Long Hall, "Biology, Sexism, and Sex Hormones in the 1920s," in *Women and*

Philosophy: Toward a Theory of Liberation, ed. Carol C. Gould and Marx W. Wartofsky (New York: Putnam, 1976), 91.

25. Roberts, *Messengers*, 38.

26. Louis Berman, *The Glands Regulating Personality: A Study of the Glands of Internal Secretion in Relation to the Types of Human Nature* (New York: Macmillan, 1922), 142; also see Bernice L. Hausman, *Changing Sex: Transsexualism, Technology, and the Idea of Gender* (Durham, NC: Duke University Press, 1995), 41.

27. Louis Berman, *The Personal Equation* (New York: Century, 1925), 252.

28. Ibid., 252.

29. Ibid.

30. Frank Lillie, "General Biological Introduction," in *Sex and Internal Secretions: A Survey of Recent Research*, ed. Edgar Allen, 2nd edition (Baltimore, MD: Williams and Wilkins, 1939), 3–4, cited in Hausman, *Changing Sex*, 39 n. 58.

31. Oudshoorn, "Endocrinologists," 185.

32. F. H. Matthews, "The Americanization of Sigmund Freud: Adaptations of Psychoanalysis before 1917," *Journal of American Studies* 1:1 (April 1967): 39–62.

33. See, e.g., Ernest Jones, *On the Nightmare* (London: Hogarth, 1931), esp. 299; Charles Berg, "The Unconscious Significance of Hair," *International Journal of Psycho-Analysis* 17 (1936): 73–88.

34. "If you reject this idea as fantastic," Freud concluded, "I am of course defenceless." Sigmund Freud, "Femininity," in *The Standard Edition of the Complete Psychological Works of Sigmund Freud*, ed. James Strachey, vol. 22 (London: Hogarth, 1953 [1933]), 132.

35. Samuel Wyllis Bandler, *The Endocrines* (Philadelphia: Saunders, 1921), iv, cited in Chandak Sengoopta, *The Most Secret Quintessence of Life: Sex, Glands, and Hormones, 1850–1950* (Chicago: University of Chicago Press, 2006), 72.

36. Hausman, *Changing Sex*, 28.

37. André Tridon, *Psychoanalysis and Gland Personalities* (New York: Brentano's, 1923), 11; Hausman, *Changing Sex*, 30.

38. Nathan G. Hale, "From Berggasse XIX to Central Park West: The Americanization of Psychoanalysis, 1919–1940," *Journal of the History of the Behavioral Sciences* 14 (1978): 30.

39. Berman, *Glands Regulating Personality*, 127.

40. Laurence H. Mayers and Arthur D. Welton, *What We Are and Why: A Study with Illustrations, of the Relation of the Endocrine Glands to Human*

Conduct and Dispositional Traits, with Special Reference to the Influence of Gland Derangements on Behavior (New York: Dodd, Mead, 1933), 26.

41. Berman, *Glands Regulating Personality*, 129, 128.

42. The term "hirsuties" predates "hirsutism" in the medical literature by several years; neither was in wide circulation until the 1930s. The *Oxford English Dictionary* lists the latter's earliest appearance as "Hirsutism and Suprarenal Virilism," *Journal of the American Medical Association*, March 19, 1927. The disease term appears to have been used in French as early as 1910. See M. Ch. Achard and J. Thiers, "Le virilisme pilaire et son association à l'insuffisance glycolytique (Diabète des femmes à barbe)," *Bulletin de l'Academie Nationale de Medecine* 86 (1921): 51, citing Apert, *Bulletin de la Société de pédiatrie* (1910).

43. A search of more than four thousand articles on hirsutism in the online database Medline limited to "hirsutism and male not female" yielded 123 results; the reverse search, for "hirsutism and female not male" produced 2,675 results. ("Male" and "female" are used as keywords to mark articles, and sometimes as a matter of course both male and female are entered, even if males are not the subject of the article. My thanks to Alison Vander Zanden for her astute observation on this point.)

44. William Alexander Newman Dorland, *American Illustrated Medical Dictionary* (Philadelphia: Saunders, 1922), 482. Dorland's defines "virilism" as the "development of masculine physical and mental traits in the female" (1168).

45. Achard and Thiers, 51–66. See also William Jeffcoate and Marie-France Kong, "*Diabète des femmes à barbe*: A Classic Paper Reread," *Lancet*, September 30, 2000, 1183–85.

46. "The Endocrine Glands—A Caution," *Journal of the American Medical Association*, May 28, 1921, 1500.

47. A superb review of these studies may be found in Joan Ferrante, "Biomedical versus Cultural Constructions of Abnormality: The Case of Idiopathic Hirsutism in the United States," *Culture, Medicine, and Psychiatry* 12 (1988): 219–38.

48. David Ferriman and J. P. Gallwey, "Clinical Assessment of Body Hair Growth in Women," *Journal of Clinical Endocrinology and Metabolism* 21:11 (1961): 1440–47.

49. Herman Goodman, "The Problem of Excess Hair," *Hygeia* 8 (May 1930): 432.

50. R. G. Hoskins, *The Tides of Life: The Endocrine Glands in Bodily Adjustment* (New York: Norton, 1933), 152.

51. Howard T. Behrman, "Diagnosis and Management of Hirsutism," *Journal of the American Medical Association*, April 23, 1960, 1924.

52. George Chauncey Jr., "Christian Brotherhood or Sexual Perversion? Homosexual Identities and the Construction of Sexual Boundaries in the World War One Era," *Journal of Social History* 19:2 (Winter 1985): 189–211; Jennifer Terry, *An American Obsession: Science, Medicine, and Homosexuality in Modern Society* (Chicago: University of Chicago Press, 1999).

53. Hausman, *Changing Sex*, 30; Kenen, "Who Counts," 200.

54. Clifford A. Wright, "Further Studies of Endocrine Aspects of Homosexuality," *Medical Record* 147 (1938): 408, cited in Sengoopta, *The Most Secret Quintessence of Life*, 317 n. 255.

55. Stafford, "Adrenal Glands," 133.

56. Max G. Schlapp and Edward H. Smith, *The New Criminology: A Consideration of the Chemical Causation of Abnormal Behavior* (New York: Boni and Liveright, 1928), 215.

57. Roberta Milliken, *Ambiguous Locks: An Iconology in Medieval Art and Literature* (London: McFarland, 2012).

58. See, e.g., Samuel Simon, *Hairfree: The Story of Electrolysis* (1948), 14. Available online at http://www.ncbi.nlm.nih.gov/pmc/articles/PMC1520635.

59. A. F. Niemoeller, *Superfluous Hair and Its Removal* (New York: Harvest House, 1938), 28.

60. Delmar Emil Bordeaux, *Cosmetic Electrolysis and the Removal of Superfluous Hair* (Rockford, IL: Bellevue, 1942), 13.

61. On the use of lesbian baiting against political activists more generally, see Cynthia Rothschild, *Written Out: How Sexuality Is Used to Attack Women's Organizing* (New York: IGLHC, 2005); Hausman, *Changing Sex*, 38.

62. Berman, *Glands Regulating Personality*, 313–29; William Wolf, *Endocrinology in Modern Practice*, 2nd edition (Philadelphia: Saunders, 1939), 22–25.

63. Roberts, *Messengers of Sex*, 36; Chandak Sengoopta, *The Most Secret Quintessence of Life: Sex, Glands, and Hormones, 1850–1950* (Chicago: University of Chicago Press, 2006), 72–73; Roy Porter and Lesley Hall, *The Facts of Life: The Creation of Sexual Knowledge in Britain, 1650–1950* (New Haven, CT: Yale University Press, 1995), esp. 175; Hausman, *Changing Sex*, 30.

64. Hoskins, *Tides of Life*, 336.

65. Edward Smith, "The Reds and the Glands," *Saturday Evening Post*, August 21, 1920, 6–7, 162, 165–66, 169–70; and Smith, "Your Emotions Will Get You If You Don't Watch Out," *American Magazine*, August 1925, 32–33, 72–74; Hausman, *Changing Sex*, 27.

66. Louis Berman, *Glands Regulating Personality*, 290–91. See also Hausman,

Changing Sex, 23; Sengoopta, *Secret Quintessence of Life*, 73.

67. Hausman, *Changing Sex*, 38.

68. Gland extracts also were used to try to make bald men *grow* hair—as when a physician at the University of Illinois College of Medicine tried injecting patients with pituitary gland extract in the late 1920s. See "Gland Extract Makes Bald Heads Grow Hair," *Popular Science*, April 1932, 43.

69. Wayne L. Whitaker and Burton L. Baker, "Inhibition of Hair Growth by Percutaneous Application of Certain Adrenal Cortical Preparations," *Science*, August 27, 1948, 207–9.

70. Schultheiss, Denil, and Jonas, "Rejuvenation," 351–55; Hoberman and Yesalis, "History of Synthetic Testosterone," 60–65; Nelly Oudshoorn, "On Measuring Sex Hormones: The Role of Biological Assays in Sexualizing Chemical Substances," *Bulletin of the History of Medicine* 64 (1990): 255.

71. See, e.g., A. Vermulen and J. C. M. Verplancke, "A Simple Method for the Determination of Urinary Testosterone Excretion in Human Urine," *Steroids* 2 (1963): 453. Bernice L. Hausman points out that the advent of noninjectables enabled users to adapt hormonal therapies to their own purposes, as pills might be exchanged or redosed "outside the supervision of professional medicine." See Hausman, *Changing Sex*, 33.

72. David Serlin, *Replaceable You: Engineering the Body in Postwar America* (Chicago: University of Chicago Press, 2004). See also Hausman, *Changing Sex*, esp. 23, 43.

73. Simon, *Hairfree*, 66–67.

74. American Medical Association Historical Health Fraud Collection, Chicago, Illinois (hereafter AMA), N. H. Franz of Urbana, Ohio, to AMA, December 19, 1931, folder 0316-06.

75. Eric E. Winter of Wilson Schools in Dayton, Ohio, to AMA, March 14, 1949, folder 0925-03, AMA.

76. Reply to Eric E. Winter, March 28, 1949, folder 0925-03, AMA.

77. Hoskins, *Tides of Life*, 340–41.

78. Arthur J. Cramp to Gordon Smith of Chicago, May 14, 1930, folder 0317-02, AMA. See also Arthur J. Cramp to Clyde I. Backus, May 14, 1930, folder 0317-02, AMA.

79. Segre, *Androgens*, 89.

80. On the role of hormone therapy in gender transitions, see Hausman, *Changing Sex*; Meyerowitz, *How Sex Changed*. One of the most common endocrine disorders associated with hirsutism, polycystic ovary syndrome (PCOS), became a prime therapeutic application; see Celia Kitzinger and Jo Willmott, "'The Thief of Womanhood': Women's Experience of Polycys-

tic Ovarian Syndrome," *Social Science & Medicine* 54 (2002): 349–61.

81. Andrée Boisselle and Roland R. Tremblay, "New Therapeutic Approach to the Hirsute Patient," *Fertility and Sterility* 32:3 (September 1979): 278.

82. Shapiro and Evron, "Novel Use of Spironolactone," 432.

83. D. Delanoe et al., "Androgenisation of Female Partners of Men on Medroxyprogesterone Acetate/Percutaneous Testosterone Contraception," *Lancet*, February 4, 1984, 276.

84. Jocelyn R. Rentoul, "Management of the Hirsute Woman," *International Journal of Dermatology* 22:5 (June 1983): 269.

85. "Hairy Legs," *British Medical Journal*, October 2, 1976, 777.

NOTES TO CHAPTER 6

1. Harriet Lyons and Rebecca Rosenblatt, "Body Hair: The Last Frontier," *Ms. Magazine*, July 1972, 64–65, 131.

2. Mary Thom, *Inside Ms.: 25 Years of the Magazine and the Feminist Movement* (New York: Holt, 1997), 53.

3. *Time* magazine described feminists as not only "strident," "humorless," and "extremist" but also "hairy legged." See Martha Fineman and Martha T. McCluskey, eds., *Feminism, Media, and the Law* (New York: Oxford University Press, 1997), 14.

4. "TV Mailbag—Dear Jane: Shave," *New York Times*, April 29, 1973, cited in Gail Collins, *When Everything Changed: The Amazing Journey of American Women from 1960 to the Present* (Little, Brown, 2009), 171.

5. Anna Quindlen, "Out of the Skyboxes," *Newsweek*, October 15, 2007, 90.

6. Thom, *Inside Ms.*, 41. Apparently Helen Gurley Brown was similarly vexed by the antishaving perspective. See Jennifer Scanlon, *Bad Girls Go Everywhere: The Life of Helen Gurley Brown* (New York: Oxford University Press, 2009), 176.

7. Betty Friedan, *It Changed My Life: Writings on the Women's Movement* (New York: Norton, 1985 [1963]), xvi.

8. Judith Hennessee, *Betty Friedan: Her Life* (New York: Random House, 1999), 184. Hennessee further notes that Friedan claimed that Steinem told other women that "they didn't have to bother to wear makeup or shave their legs," but in actuality (Hennessee reports) "neither Gloria nor *Ms.* told other women not to look good" (161). Hennessee further claims that the revised introduction to Friedan's best-selling book lambasts *Ms.* for "encouraging women to throw away their razors and stop shaving under their arms" (184): "Like Gloria (and virtually everyone else in public life with

an image to protect), Betty had a tendency to rewrite history. *Ms.* had no policy on hair" (184).

9. On the "second wave," see Marsha Lear, "The Second Feminist Wave," *New York Times Magazine*, March 10, 1968, 24–25, 50, 53, 55–56, 58, 60, 62; Maggie Humm, *The Dictionary of Feminist Theory* (Columbus: Ohio State University Press, 1990), 198. On hair, specifically, see Rachel Blau DuPlessis and Ann Snitow, eds., *The Feminist Memoir Project* (New York: Three Rivers Press, 1998), 166; Nancy Whittier, *Feminist Generations: The Persistence of the Radical Women's Movement* (Philadelphia: Temple University Press, 1995), 144.

10. See, for instance, Carolyn Mackler, "Memoirs of a (Sorta) Ex-Shaver," in *Body Outlaws: Young Women Write about Body Image and Identity*, ed. Ophira Edut (Seattle: Seal Press, 2000), 55–61; Jennifer Margulis, "Musings on Hairy Legs," *Sojourner* 20:8 (April 1995): 9, 11.

11. "Julia Roberts, Uncovered," *Ottawa Citizen*, May 1, 1999; "Her Personality's the Pits!" *Newsweek*, July 23, 2001.

12. See, e.g., Catherine Saint Louis, "Unshaven Women: Free Spirits or Unkempt?" *New York Times*, April 12, 2010; "Leg Work: Body Hair Is Not Always a Statement," *Jezebel*, April 13, 2010, http://jezebel.com/5516049/leg-work-body-hair-is-not-always-a-statement.

13. "Feminism isn't always pretty (see: underarm hair). Without it, however, Kate O'Beirne would have been unlikely to have this book published—and most women would not have their own money to waste on it." Ana Marie Cox, "Easy Targets: A *National Review* Editor Revisits the Excesses of Feminism" [review of Kate O'Beirne, *Women Who Make the World Worse and How Their Radical Feminist Assault Is Ruining Our Families, Military, Schools, and Sports*], *New York Times Book Review*, Sunday, January 15, 2006, 21.

14. J. J. Perret, *La Pogonotomie, ou L'Art D'Apprendre A Se Raser Soi-Meme* (Yverdon, 1770).

15. Russell B. Adams Jr., *King C. Gillette: The Man and His Wonderful Shaving Device* (Boston: Little, Brown, 1978), 26–46.

16. Richard L. Bushman and Claudia L. Bushman, "The Early History of Cleanliness in America," *Journal of American History* 74:4 (March 1988): 1214.

17. Thomas J. Schlereth, "Conduits and Conduct: Home Utilities in Victorian America, 1876–1915," in *American Home Life, 1880–1930: A Social History of Spaces and Services*, ed. Jessica H. Foy and Thomas J. Schlereth (Knoxville: University of Tennessee Press, 1992), 226; Martin V. Melosi, *The Sanitary*

City: Urban Infrastructure in America from Colonial Times to the Present (Baltimore, MD: Johns Hopkins University Press, 2000), 22, 30.

18. Katherine Ashenburg, *The Dirt on Clean: An Unsanitized History* (New York: North Point Press, 2007), 224, 236; Maureen Ogle, *All the Modern Conveniences: American Household Plumbing, 1840–1890* (Baltimore, MD: Johns Hopkins University Press, 1996).

19. Elizabeth Shove, *Comfort, Cleanliness, and Convenience: The Social Organization of Normality* (Oxford: Berg, 2003), 106; Ogle, *Modern Conveniences*; Marina Moskowitz, *Standard of Living: The Measure of the Middle Class in Modern America* (Baltimore, MD: Johns Hopkins University Press, 2004), chap. 2.

20. Quoted in Shove, *Comfort*, 101; Nancy Tomes, *The Gospel of Germs: Men, Women, and the Microbe in American Life* (Cambridge, MA: Harvard University Press, 1998); Bushman and Bushman, "Early History," 1213; Suellen M. Hoy, *Chasing Dirt: The American Pursuit of Cleanliness* (New York: Oxford University Press, 1995).

21. Ashenburg, *Dirt on Clean*, 207, 219; Carroll W. Purcell, *The Machine in America: A Social History of Technology* (Baltimore, MD: Johns Hopkins University Press, 1995), 249.

22. Ashenburg, *Dirt on Clean*, 224.

23. Mark Pendergast, *Mirror Mirror: A History of the Human Love Affair with Reflection* (New York: Basic Books, 2003); Sabine Bonnet, *The Mirror: A History*, trans. Katharine H. Jewett (New York: Routledge, 2001).

24. Ashenburg, *Dirt on Clean*, 220.

25. Shove, *Comfort*, 79; Schlereth, "Conduits and Conduct," 238.

26. Adams, *King C. Gillette*, 101.

27. G. Bruce Retallack, "Razors, Shaving, and Gender Construction: An Inquiry into the Material Culture of Shaving," *Material History Review* 49 (Spring 1999): 8; Adams, *King C. Gillette*, 102.

28. *Life*, May 17, 1917, 875.

29. *Outlook*, May 16, 1917, 117.

30. Adams, *King C. Gillette*, 104.

31. Retallack, "Razors," 8; Adams, *King C. Gillette*, 96–105.

32. Retallack, "Razors," 6.

33. See the Gillette advertisement in *Life*, June 3, 1915, 1009. Also see van Oost, "Materialized Gender," 202.

34. "Advice for Women Who Shave," *Today's Health*, July 1964, 50.

35. Jeffrey L. Meikle, *American Plastic: A Cultural History* (New Brunswick, NJ: Rutgers University Press, 1995), 137. Meikle further notes that nylon

stockings were in short supply even before the United States entered the war, as consumers impatiently scrambled to scoop up Du Pont's "run proof stockings" at $1.15 a pair, while industry leaders, fretful about the prospect of "stockings that would last forever," did little to increase manufacturing capacity (146).

36. Meikle, *American Plastic*, 147; "Opaque Leg," *Fortune*, October 1942, 26, 30; "Stockings Scarce," *Business Week*, March 3, 1945, 90.

37. "Opaque Leg," *Fortune*, 30; "Less Leg Lure," *Business Week*, November 7, 1942, 64. The Office of Price Administration set a nationwide ceiling on hosiery prices ($1.65) in response to the shortage.

38. "Bottled 'Stockings,'" *Consumer Reports*, July 1943, 181.

39. Ibid., 181.

40. "Cosmetic Stockings," *Consumer Reports*, July 1944, 172.

41. Ibid., 172; "Bottled 'Stockings,'" *Consumer Reports*, 181.

42. "Cosmetic Stockings," *Consumer Reports*, 172. See also Edith Efron, "Legs Are Bare Because They Can't Be Sheer," *New York Times Magazine*, June 24, 1945, 17.

43. "Instead of Stockings," *Consumer Reports*, July 1945, 175.

44. Gerald Wendt, "Reports on Products: Stockings from a Bottle," *Consumer Reports*, August 1942, 202; "Stocking Savers & Substitutes," *Consumer Reports*, September 1941, 138–39; "Cosmetic Stockings," *Consumer Reports*, 172–74; Richard Polenberg, *War and Society: The United States, 1941–1945* (New York: Lippincott, 1972), 8–11; "Advice for Women Who Shave," *Today's Health*, July 1964, 37.

45. Thomas Hine, *Populuxe* (New York: Knopf, 1986), 66; Anthony L. Andrady, ed., *Plastics and the Environment* (Hoboken, NJ: Wiley, 2003), 33–36; Retallack, "Razors," 9.

46. bell hooks, *Killing Rage* (New York: Holt, 1995), 122, 120.

47. Tracey Owens Patton, "'Hey Girl, Am I More Than My Hair?' African American Women and Their Struggles with Beauty, Body Image, and Hair," *NWSA Journal* 18:2 (Summer 2006): 40; hooks, "Black Beauty and Black Power," in *Killing Rage*, 119–32.

48. Dominick Cavallo, cited in Gael Graham, "Flaunting the Freak Flag: *Karr v. Schmidt* and the Great Hair Debate in American High Schools, 1965–1975," *Journal of American History* 91:2 (2004): 541. See also Anthony Synnott, *The Body Social: Symbolism, Self, and Society* (London: Routledge, 1993), 115–16; Mary Douglas, *Natural Symbols* (Harmondsworth, England: Pelican, 1973 [1970]), 102.

49. David Allyn, *Make Love, Not War: The Sexual Revolution, an Unfettered*

History (Boston: Little, Brown, 2000), 125–26.

50. Alexander Bloom and Wini Breines, eds., *"Takin' It to the Streets": A Sixties Reader* (New York: Oxford University Press, 1995), 459–557; Sara Evans, *Personal Politics: The Roots of Women's Liberation in the Civil Rights Movement and New Left* (New York: Vintage, 1980 [1979]); Robin Morgan, ed., *Sisterhood Is Powerful: An Anthology of Writings from the Women's Liberation Movement* (New York: Vintage, 1970); Alice Echols, *Daring to Be Bad: Radical Feminism in America, 1967–1975* (Minneapolis: University of Minnesota Press, 1989); Karen Anderson, *Changing Woman: A History of Racial Ethnic Women in Modern America* (New York: Oxford University Press, 1996); Gabriela F. Arredondo, ed., *Chicana Feminisms: A Critical Reader* (Durham, NC: Duke University Press, 2003); Lillian Faderman, *Odd Girls and Twilight Lovers: A History of Lesbian Life in Twentieth-Century America* (New York: Penguin, 1991); Stephanie Gilmore, ed., *Feminist Coalitions: Historical Perspectives on Second-Wave Feminism in the United States* (Urbana: University of Illinois Press, 2008).

51. Cited in Evans, *Personal Politics*, 212.

52. Cited in Eric Foner, *The Story of American Freedom* (New York: Norton, 1998), 295.

53. Heywood cited in Rosalind Pollack Petchesky, "Reproductive Freedom: Beyond 'A Woman's Right to Choose,'" *Signs* 5:4 (1980): 666.

54. Sandra Morgen, *Into Our Own Hands: The Women's Health Movement in the United States, 1969–1990* (New Brunswick, NJ: Rutgers University Press, 2002), 17–22; Kathy Davis, *The Making of* Our Bodies, Ourselves: *How Feminism Travels across Borders* (Durham, NC: Duke University Press, 2007); Michelle Murphy, "Liberation through Control in the Body Politics of U.S. Radical Feminism," in *The Moral Authority of Nature*, ed. Lorraine Daston and Fernando Vidal (Chicago: University of Chicago Press, 2004), 331–55; and idem, *Seizing the Means of Reproduction: Entanglements of Feminism, Health, and Technoscience* (Durham, NC: Duke University Press, 2012), esp. 87–88.

55. See Robbie E. Davis-Floyd's thorough discussion in *Birth as an American Rite of Passage* (Berkeley: University of California Press, 2003 [1992]), 83–84. Physicians' public discussion of the merits (or lack thereof) of obstetrical shaving began several years before critics of technocratic hospital births took up the cause. See, e.g., W. J. Sweeney, "Perineal Shaves and Bladder Catheterizations: Necessary and Benign, or Unnecessary and Potentially Injurious?" *Obstetrics and Gynecology* 21 (1963): 291; H. I. Kantor et al., "Value of Shaving the Pudendal-Perineal Area in Delivery Preparation,"

Obstetrics and Gynecology 25 (1965): 509; R. L. Nooyen, "Removal of Pubic Hair for Delivery without Shaving," *Journal of the American Osteopathic Association* 66:1 (1966): 58; and A. E. Long, "The Unshaved Perineum at Parturition: A Bacteriologic Study," *American Journal of Obstetrics and Gynecology* 99:3 (1967): 333.

56. Joanne Meyerowitz, *How Sex Changed: A History of Transsexuality in the United States* (Cambridge, MA: Harvard University Press, 2002), 247.

57. Robin Morgan, *Going Too Far: The Personal Chronicle of a Feminist* (New York: Random House, 1977 [1968]), 108, 107.

58. Cited in Synnott, *Body Social*, 119.

59. Germaine Greer, *The Female Eunuch* (New York: McGraw-Hill, 1971 [1970]), 28.

60. Lyons and Rosenblatt, "Body Hair," 131.

61. Ibid., 131.

62. "Six Ways to Get Rid of Unwanted Hair," *Good Housekeeping*, July 1978, 244; "Removing Unwanted Hair Permanently, Not a Do-It-Yourself Job," *Consumer Bulletin*, October 1966, 34–36; "Hair You Don't Want," *Harper's Bazaar*, April 1974, 43; "Hair That You Can Do Without," *Vogue*, April 15, 1970, 121–22. For further discussion of how second-wave feminisms were co-opted as "new strategies of market segmentation," see Lizabeth Cohen, *A Consumer's Republic: The Politics of Mass Consumption in Postwar America* (New York: Vintage, 2003), 316; Susan J. Douglas, "Narcissism as Liberation," in *The Gender and Consumer Culture Reader*, ed, Jennifer Scanlon (New York: New York University Press, 2000), 267–82.

63. "Employee Harassed by 'Hairy Legs' Insult and Touching," *Federal Human Resources Week*. December 21, 1998: *Frantaga C. Humphrey v. Henderson, Postmaster General, U.S. Postal Service*, 99 FEOR 3090 (EEOC Comm. 10/16/98).

64. *Built Like That* (Subtle Sister Productions), 2001.

65. Available at http://radcheers.tripod.com/RC/id1.html. Thanks to S. Stone and Hannah Johnson-Breimeier for bringing the cheer to my attention.

66. A LexisNexis search of major U.S. publications reveals a more than six-fold increase in references to "bearded terrorists" in the two years following the attacks of September 11, 2001, as compared to the two years beginning September 1999.

67. See "Freedom in Peril: Guarding the 2nd Amendment in the 21st Century," 2006, available at http://boingboing.net/images/NR-F8_PERILFINAL. pdf; Marcus Baram, "NRA's Graphic Attack on Its Enemies Leaked onto Internet," *ABC News*, December 29, 2006, http://abcnews.go.com/US/

story?id=2759754; "Is This (Freedom in Peril) an Actual NRA Document?" *AR15.com: Home of the Black Rifle Archive Server,* December 27–31, 2006, http://www.ar15.com/archive/topic.html?b=1&f=5&t=530989.
There is a certain irony in the NRA's association of hairiness and animal rights, given that strong words have been exchanged between the heads of People for the Ethical Treatment of Animals and the National Organization for Women over hair removal: NOW accused PETA of misogyny for an ad that seemed to describe female pubic hair as disgusting. See "Crossing the Bikini Line," *Harper's Magazine,* April 2000, 26–28; "Fur, Smoothed," *Harper's Magazine,* June 2000, 18–20.

68. Murphy, "Liberation," 352; Foner, *Story of American Freedom,* 295.

NOTES TO CHAPTER 7

1. See "Sex and Another City," September 17, 2000 (*Sex and the City,* season 3, episode 14).

2. Debra Herbenik et al., "Pubic Hair Removal among Women in the United States: Prevalence, Methods, and Characteristics," *Journal of Sexual Medicine* 7 (2010): 3322–30.

3. Michael Boroughs et al., "'Male Depilation' Prevalence and Associated Features of Body Hair Removal," *Sex Roles* 52 (2005): 637–44; Matthew Immergut, "Manscaping: The Tangle of Nature, Culture, and Male Body Hair," in *The Body Reader: Essential Social and Cultural Readings,* ed. Lisa Jean Moore and Mary Kosut (New York: New York University Press, 2010), 287–304.

4. See, for example, the case of a 25-year-old bride whose pubic hair was so matted as to render coition on the first night of marriage "impracticable." Physicians resolved the problem with a paste composed of arsenic, copper sulfate, lime, soap, and water. See "Pathology," *North American Medical and Surgical Journal* 12 (October 1831): 455.

5. Sarah Hildebrandt, "The Last Frontier: Body Norms and Hair Removal Practices in Contemporary American Culture," in *The EmBodyment of American Culture,* ed. Heinz Tschachler, Maureen Devine, and Michael Draxlbauer (Munich: Lit Verlag, 2003), 59–71.

6. Ruth Barcan, *Nudity: A Cultural Anatomy* (Oxford: Berg, 2004), 148; Wendy Cooper, *Hair: Sex, Society, Symbolism* (London: Aldus, 1971), 116, 89.

7. Lenore Riddell, Hannah Varto, and Zoe Hodgson, "Smooth Talking: The Phenomenon of Pubic Hair Removal in Women," *Canadian Journal of Hu-*

man Sexuality, 19 (2010): 121–30; Jonathan D. K. Trager, "Pubic Hair Removal: Pearls and Pitfalls," *Journal of Pediatric and Adolescent Gynecology* 19 (2006): 117.

8. Kristin Tillotson, "Liberation Gone Wild: Is This Power and Freedom or a Post-Feminist Backslide?" *Star Tribune* (Minneapolis, Minnesota), December 18, 2005, 1F.

9. Ariel Levy, *Female Chauvinist Pigs: Women and the Rise of Raunch Culture* (New York: Free Press, 2005), 4.

10. Sheila Jeffreys, *Beauty and Misogyny: Harmful Cultural Practices in the West* (London: Routledge, 2005), 4. Other analysts take a similarly dour view of genital depilation, seeing in it an intensification of social control of the female body in general and the construction of women as childlike and "powerless" in particular. See, e.g., Marika Tiggeman and Sarah J. Kenyon, "The Hairless Norm: The Removal of Body Hair in Women," *Sex Roles* 39 (1998): 874; Susan A. Basow, "The Hairless Ideal: Women and Their Body Hair," *Psychology of Women Quarterly* 15 (1991): 83–96; Susan Brownmiller, *Femininity* (London: Hamish Hamilton, 1984); Christine Hope, "Caucasian Female Body Hair and American Culture," *Journal of American Culture* 5 (1982): 93–99; Magdala Peixoto Labre, "The Brazilian Wax: New Hairlessness Norm for Women?" *Journal of Communication Inquiry* 26 (2002): 113–32; Sarita Srivastava, "'Unwanted Hair Problem?' Struggling to Re-Present Our Bodies," *Rungh: A South Asian Quarterly of Culture, Comment, and Criticism* 1:4 (1993): 5–7.

11. Kira Cochrane, "A Choice Too Far," *New Statesman*, September 24, 2007, 30–31.

12. Ibid., 30–31.

13. Rex W. Huppke, "Brazilian Wax Ban in New Jersey Is Scrapped," *Chicago Tribune*, March 21, 2009, http://archives.chicagotribune.com/2009/mar/21/news/chi-talk-bikiniwax-0321mar21.

14. Mimi Spencer, "Freedom Is a Hairy Body," *Age*, February 24, 2003, http://www.theage.com.au/articles/2003/02/23/1045935277714.html.

15. Jennifer Baumgardner and Amy Richards, *Manifesta: Young Women, Feminism, and the Future* (New York: Farrar, Straus, Giroux, 2000), 56–57 (emphasis in original).

16. Cochrane, "Choice," 30–31.

17. Labre, "Brazilian Wax," 121, 117. Also see Janea Padhila with Martha Frankel, *Brazilian Sexy: Secrets to Living a Gorgeous and Confident Life* (New York: Penguin, 2010).

18. See Liddell, Varto, and Hodgson, "Smooth Talking."

19. As complete genital depilation was routinized, salons began to experiment with ways to continue to entice high-end, specialty clientele. A brief fervor for fox merkins, tiny fur patches worn over the depilated pubic region, reflects this effort. See http://www.dailymail.co.uk/femail/article-2093860/Cindy-Barshops-fox-fur-merkins-given-faux-makeover-PETA-claims-victory-bizarre-beauty-fad.html.

20. Christina Valhouli, "Faster Pussycat, Wax! Wax!" *Salon.com*, September 3, 1999.

21. Trager, "Pubic Hair Removal," 118; Sara Ramsey et al., "Pubic Hair and Sexuality: A Review," *Journal of Sexual Medicine* 6 (2009): 2106; Hank Stuever, "Mr. Rug: For Men, a Hairy Back Is a Closely Held Secret," *Washington Post*, August 3, 2000; Olivia Barker, "The Male Resistance to Waxing Is Melting Away," *USA Today*, August 23, 2005.

22. See Joanne Meyerowitz's excellent discussion of this longer trajectory, "Women, Cheesecake, and Borderline Material: Responses to Girlie Pictures in the Mid-Twentieth-Century U.S.," *Journal of Women's History* 8:3 (Fall 1996): 9–35.

23. See Paul R. Abramson, Steven D. Pinkerton, Mark Huppin, *Sexual Rights in America: The Ninth Amendment and the Pursuit of Happiness* (New York: New York University Press, 2003); Jack Hafferkamp, "Un-Banning Books: How the Courts of the United States Came to Extend First Amendment Guarantees to Include Pornography," in *Porn 101: Eroticism, Pornography, and the First Amendment*, ed. James Elias et al. (Amherst, NY: Prometheus, 1999), 396–413.

24. The relaxation of pornography regulation also coincided with an important technical shift: the rise of the sixteen-millimeter film. Film historian Eric Schaeffer notes that the popularity of sixteen-millimeter film gauge stemmed in part from its wide use in World War II newsreel and combat photography. After the war, the film gauge was picked up by film students and soon came to be associated with the wider waves of dissent sweeping college campuses. The relative affordability of sixteen-millimeter film provoked cinematic experimentation, including in pornographic film. By the midseventies, the feature-length, x-rated film had largely supplanted the silent, illegally produced and displayed "stag" picture. See Eric Schaeffer, "Gauging a Revolution: 16 mm Film and the Rise of the Pornographic Feature," in *Porn Studies*, ed. Linda Williams (Durham, NC: Duke University Press, 2004), 393, 375–76. Also see Luke Ford, *A History of X: 100 Years*

of Sex in Film (Amherst, NY: Prometheus, 1999), 37.

25. Ford, *History of X*, 30.

26. Schaeffer, "Gauging a Revolution," 376–78, 381, 394 n. 1; see also Linda Williams, *Hard Core: Power, Pleasure, and the "Frenzy of the Visible"* (Berkeley: University of California Press, 1999), 96–97; Justin Wyatt, "The Stigma of X: Adult Cinema and the Institution of the MPAA Rating System," in *Controlling Hollywood: Censorship and Regulation in the Studio Era*, ed. Matthew Bernstein (New Brunswick, NJ: Rutgers University Press, 1999); Jon Lewis, *Hollywood v. Hard Core: How the Struggle over Censorship Saved the Modern Film Industry* (New York: New York University Press, 2000); Ford, *History of X*, 30–41. It might be noted in this context that the former all-female Beaver College changed its name to Arcadia University in 2001, both to sever ties to its single-sex history and to avoid crude jokes. See Alan Finder, "To Woo Students, Colleges Choose Names That Sell," *New York Times*, August 11, 2005.

27. Joseph P. Slade, "Pornographic Theaters Off Times Square," in *The Pornography Controversy: Changing Moral Standards in American Life*, ed. Ray C. Rist (New Brunswick, NJ: Transaction, 1975), 123. For further reflection on the cultural and economic connections between women and fur, see Chantal Nadeau, "'My Furladies': The Fabric of a Nation," in *Thinking through the Skin*, ed. Sara Ahmed and Jackie Stacey (London: Routledge, 2001), 194–208.

28. David Allyn, *Make Love, Not War: The Sexual Revolution, an Unfettered History* (Boston: Little, Brown, 2000), 285, 287.

29. Harriet Lyons and Rebecca Rosenblatt, "Body Hair: The Last Frontier," *Ms. Magazine*, July 1972, 64–65, 131.

30. Vanessa R. Schick et al., "Evulvalution: The Portrayal of Women's External Genitalis and Physique across Time and the Current Barbie Doll Ideals," *Journal of Sex Research* 47 (2010): 1–9; Ros Bramwell, "Invisible Labia: The Representation of Female External Genitals in Women's Magazines," *Sexual and Relationship Therapy* 17 (2002): 187–190.

31. Ramsey et al., "Pubic Hair," 2105. This claim neglects "bear"-themed porn, devoted to depictions of large, hairy men. On bear communities and their impressive defiance of hairless norms, see Ron Jackson Suresha, *Bears on Bears: Interviews and Discussions* (Los Angeles: Alyson Books, 2002).

32. Ramsey et al., 2105. Correlations also have been established more generally between women's consumption of fashion magazines and popular television programs and the frequency and amount of pubic hair removed. See Marika Tiggemann and Suzanna Hodgson, "The Hairlessness Norm Ex-

tended: Reasons for and Predictors of Women's Body Hair Removal at Different Body Sites," *Sex Roles* 59:11 (2008): 889-97.

33. Susann Cokal, "Clean Porn: The Visual Aesthetics of Hygiene, Hot Sex, and Hair Removal," *Pop-Porn: Pornography in American Culture*, ed. Ann C. Hall and Mardia J. Bishop (Westport, CT: Praeger, 2007); Barcan, *Nudity*, 28.

34. Cooper, *Hair*; Victoria Sherrow, *For Appearance' Sake: The Historical Encyclopedia of Good Looks, Beauty, and Grooming* (Phoenix, AZ: Oryx, 2001), 53.

35. Benjamin Godfrey, *Diseases of Hair: A Popular Treatise upon the Affections of the Hair System* (London: Churchill, 1872); Henri C. Leonard, *The Hair: Its Growth, Care, Diseases, and Treatment* (Detroit, MI: C. Henri Leonard, Medical Book Publisher, 1880); "Cosmetic Depilation," *Journal of the American Medical Association* 82 (1924): 1575; Duncan L. Buckley, "Clinical Illustrations of Diseases of the Skin," *Archives of Dermatology* 7 (1881): 149-62.

36. "Zip—Special Data, 1917–1941," American Medical Association Historical Health Fraud Collection, Chicago, Illinois, folder 0924-16.

37. Dannia Tashir and Barry Leshin, "Sugaring: An Ancient Method of Hair Removal," *Dermatologic Surgery* 27:3 (2001): 309-11.

38. P. H. Frankel, *Essentials of Petroleum: A Key to Oil Economics* (New York: Kelley, 1969); Matthew Yeomens, *Oil: Anatomy of an Industry* (New York: New Press, 2004); Toyin Falola and Ann Genova, *The Politics of the Global Oil Industry: An Introduction* (London: Praeger, 2005); International Group Inc., "Wax Refining," *IGI Wax*, 2008, http://www.igiwax.com/resource/Wax_Refining.

39. Doris de Guzman, "Demand for Natural Wax Increases," *Icis.com*, August 2008, http://www.icis.com/Articles/2008/08/18/9149059/demand-for-natural-wax-increases.html; also see Grace Beckett, "Carnauba Wax in the United States: Brazilian Foreign Trade," *Economic Geography* 19 (1945): 428-30.

40. Gwen Kay, *Dying to Be Beautiful: The Campaign for Safe Cosmetics* (Columbus: Ohio State University Press, 2005); Fran Hawthorne, *Inside the FDA: The Business and Politics behind the Drugs We Take and the Food We Eat* (Hoboken, NJ: Wiley, 2005).

41. J. Elaine Spear, "American International Industries: Zvi Ryzman's Multifaceted Company Celebrates its 35th Year," *Beauty Store Business* (June 2006), http://www.docstoc.com/docs/35513566/American-International-Industries. Several other popular plant-based hair removers, such as Nad's hair-

removing gel, are promoted as alternatives to waxing. Like waxes, however, these hair removers essentially yank hair from the body with the aid of gluey compounds.

42. Thomas M. Stanbeck et al., *Services: The New Economy* (Totowa, NJ: Allanheld, Osmun, 1981); Sven Illeris, *The Service Economy: A Geographical Approach* (Chichester, England: Wiley, 1996).

43. "North American Industry Classification System 8121 Personal Care Services," *U.S. Census Bureau*, 2002, http://www.census.gov/econ/census02/data/industry/E8121.htm.

44. "Pots of Promise: The Beauty Business," *Economist*, May 22, 2003, 69–71.

45. Market researchers stress the importance of recruiting young people to hair removal, as the nation's aging population portends a downturn in sales of hair removing products and services. See Mintel International Group, *Shaving and Hair Removal Products: May 2008* (Chicago: Mintel International Group Limited, 2008), 61.

46. Using the Google Ngram Viewer.

47. S. B. Verma, "Eyebrow Threading: A Popular Hair-Removal Procedure and Its Seldom-Discussed Complications," *Clinical and Experimental Dermatology* 34:3 (2009): 363–65; J. Litak et al., "Eyebrow Epilation by Threading: An Increasingly Popular Procedure with Some Less-Popular Outcomes; A Comprehensive Review," *Dermatologic Surgery* 37:7 (2011): 1051–54; M. Abdel-Gawad et al., "Khite: A Non-Western Technique for Temporary Hair Removal," *International Journal of Dermatology* 36:3 (1997): 217.

48. William Boyd, "Making Meat: Science, Technology, and American Poultry Production," *Technology and Culture* 42 (2001): 631–64.

49. Helen R. Bickmore, *Milady's Hair Removal Techniques: A Comprehensive Manual* (Clifton Park, NY: Delmar, 2004), 92–94.

50. Rachel Johnson, "Bush Wacked," *Spectator*, May 18, 2002, 29–30; Marina Galperina, "Bedazzled Vaginas Girl Style Now?" *Animal*, July 6, 2012, http://animalnewyork.com/2012/bedazzled-vaginas-girl-style-now-nsfw.

51. Virginia Smith, *Clean: A History of Personal Hygiene and Purity* (Oxford: Oxford University Press, 2007), 339.

52. Pierrette Hondagneu-Sotelo, *Domestica: Immigrant Workers Cleaning and Caring in the Shadows of Affluence* (Berkeley: University of California Press, 2001); Chandra Talpade Mohanty, "Women Workers and Capitalist Scripts: Ideologies of Domination, Common Interest, and the Politics of Solidarity," in *Feminist Genealogies, Colonial Legacies, Democratic Futures*, ed. M. Jacqui Alexander and Chandra Talapade Mohanty (New York:

Routledge, 1997); Kathi Weeks, "Life Within and Against Work: Affective Labor, Feminist Critique, and Post-Fordist Politics," *Ephemera: Theory and Politics in Organization* 7 (2007): 233–49; Melinda Cooper and Catherine Waldby, *Clinical Labor: Tissue Donors and Research Subjects in the Global Bioeconomy* (Durham, NC: Duke University Press, 2014).

53. Pamela Sitt, "Taking It All Off," *Seattle Times*, July 9, 2003.

54. Bickmore, *Milady's*, 60; R. F. Wagner Jr., "Medical and Technical Issues in Office Electrolysis and Thermolysis," *Journal of Dermatologic Surgery and Oncology* 19 (1993), 575–77; R. N. Richards and G. E. Meharg, *Cosmetic and Medical Electrolysis and Temporary Hair Removal: A Practice Manual and Reference Guide,* 2nd ed. (Toronto: Medric, 1997); Deborah A. Sullivan, *Cosmetic Surgery: The Cutting Edge of Commercial Medicine in America* (New Brunswick, NJ: Rutgers University Press, 2001), 192–93; Donald W. Shenenberger and Lynn M. Utecht, "Removal of Unwanted Facial Hair," *American Family Physician* 66 (2002): 1907.

55. Bickmore, *Milady's*; "North American Industry," 2002.

56. See, e.g., Jed Lipinski, "Why I Got the Male Brazilian Wax," *Salon.com*, August 19, 2010.

57. Miliann Kang, "The Managed Hand: The Commercialization of Bodies and Emotions in Korean Immigrant-Owned Nail Salons," *Gender & Society* 17 (2003): 823. See also Helene M. Lawson, "Working on Hair," *Qualitative Sociology* 22:3 (1999): 235–57.

58. Hannah McCouch, "What Your Bikini Waxer Really Thinks: A Woman Who Spends Her Days Doing Brazilian-Style Hair Removal Breaks Her Code of Silence," *Cosmopolitan*, January 2002, 91.

59. Sharon Krum, "Real Women Don't Wear Fur: The 'Brazilian' Bikini Wax Is Taking New York by Storm—But It's Not for the Faint-Hearted," *Independent* (London), November 29, 1998, 2; see also R. C. Wright, "Traumatic Folliculitis of the Legs: A Persistent Case Associated with Use of a Home Epilating Device," *Journal of the American Academy of Dermatology* 27 (5 Pt 1) (1992): 771–72.

60. See "A Waxing Waltz," http://www.youtube.com/watch?v=TY1fn6IXnjQ.

61. Bickmore, *Milady's*, 93.

62. Emily Nussbaum, "A Stranger's Touch," *New York Magazine*, November 25, 2007.

63. Even when the service workers tasked with hair removal in popular films do not speak with stereotypical "ethnic" and/or regional accents, they are portrayed by women of color. See, for example, the waxing scene in the 2005 romantic comedy, *Hitch*.

64. Here as elsewhere, contact with the most marginal and abject spheres of human society—the crotches and anuses of the body politic—falls to those assigned by race, gender, class, and citizenship to low social rank. See Charles W. Mills, "Black Trash" in *Faces of Environmental Racism: Confronting Issues of Social Justice*, ed. Laura Westra and Bill E. Lawson (Lanham, MD: Rowman and Littlefield, 2001); Richard Dyer, *White* (New York: Routledge, 1997), 39, 45; Smith, *Clean*, 15; Melissa W. Wright, *Disposable Women and Other Myths of Global Capitalism* (New York: Routledge, 2006); Saskia Sassen, "Global Cities and Survival Circuits," in *Global Woman: Nannies, Maids, and Sex Workers in the New Economy*, ed. Barbara Ehrenreich and Arlie Russell Hochschild (New York: Metropolitan, 2003).

65. See Zygmunt Bauman, *Wasted Lives: Modernity and Its Outcasts* (Malden, MA: Polity, 2004), 22–23, 15.

66. Christopher Hitchens, "On the Limits of Self-Improvement, Part II," *Vanity Fair*, December 2007; "Believe Me, It's Torture," *Vanity Fair*, August 2008.

NOTES TO CHAPTER 8

1. Howard Bargman, "Counterpoint Laser Hair Removal," *Journal of Cutaneous Medicine and Surgery* 3:5 (1991): 241.

2. Kathleen Doheny, "Just Say Zap: Lasers Take Unwanted Hair Right Off—but Not in Time for Summer," *Los Angeles Times*, May 25, 1995, E10; Melissa H. Hunter and Peter J. Carek, "Evaluation and Treatment of Women with Hirsutism," *American Family Physician*, June 15, 2003, 2565–72; C. C. Dierickx, "Hair Removal by Lasers and Intense Pulsed Light Sources," *Seminars in Cutaneous Medicine and Surgery* 19 (2000): 267–75; C. C. Dierickx, M. B. Alora, and J. S. Dover, "A Clinical Overview of Hair Removal Using Lasers and Light Sources," *Dermatologic Clinic* 17 (1999): 357–66.

3. L. Goldman et al., "Pathology of the Effect of the Laser Beam on the Skin," *Nature*, March 2, 1963, 912; L. Goldman and P. Hornby, "Radiation from a Q-switched Ruby Laser," *Journal of Investigative Dermatology* 44 (1965): 69.

4. See "Hair: Treatment Areas," *Hair Removal Journal*, http://www.hairremovaljournal.org.

5. "11.5 Million Cosmetic Procedures in 2005," News Release, *American Society for Aesthetic Plastic Surgery*, February 24, 2006, http://www.surgery.org/press/news-print.php?iid=429&section; Theresamarie Mantese et al., "Cosmetic Surgery and Informed Consent: Legal and Ethical Considerations," *Michigan Bar Journal* 85:1 (2006): 26–29.

6. "Company News: Thermolase Surges on Approval of Hair-Removal Laser," *New York Times*, April 18, 1995, D4.

7. "Hot Growth: Sizzling Companies to Watch," *Business Week*, June 5, 2006, http://www.businessweek/com/hot_growth/2006/index.html.

8. "Cosmetic Surgery Products to 2007: Market Size, Market Share, Market Leaders, Demand Forecast, and Sales," Study # 1741, *Freedonia Group*, 2004, http://www.freedoniagroup.com/Cosmetic-Surgery-Products.html.

9. Participant I, interview with author, September 3, 2009. Between 2008 and 2012, I conducted several dozen semi-structured interviews with various hair removal specialists. All interview material incorporated in the text is reported anonymously, in accordance with Bates College Institutional Review Board stipulations.

10. Participant I, interview with author, September 3, 2009; Kathy Kincade, "Alexandrite: The Unsung Hero of Hair Removal," *Laser Focus World*, 199a, 63–64, available online; Human Rights Watch Arms Project, "Blinding Laser Weapons: The Need to Ban a Cruel and Inhumane Weapon," *Human Rights Watch* 7:1 (September 1995); Human Rights Watch Arms Project, "U.S. Blinding Laser Weapons," *Human Rights Watch* 7:5 (May 1995); Joop M. Grevelink et al., "Lasers in Dermatology," *Fitzpatrick's Dermatology in General Medicine*, 5th edition, vol. 2, ed. Irwin M. Freedberg et al. (New York: McGraw Hill, 1999): 2901–21.

11. L. L. Polla et al., "Melanosomes Are a Primary Target of Q-Switched Ruby Laser Irradiation in Guinea Pig Skin," *Journal of Investigative Dermatology* 89:3 (September 1987): 281–86; A. K. Kurban et al., "Pulse Duration Effects on Cutaneous Pigment," *Lasers in Surgery and Medicine* 12:3 (1992): 282–87; K. A. Sherwood et al., "Effect of Wavelength on Cutaneous Pigment Using Pulsed Irradiation," *Journal of Investigative Dermatology* 92:5 (May 1989): 717–20; E. M. Procaccini et al., "The Effects of a Diode Laser (810nm) on Pigmented Guinea-Pig Skin," *Lasers in Medical Science* 16:3 (2001): 171–75; R. E. Fitzpatrick et al., "Pulsed Carbon Dioxide Laser, Trichloroacetic Acid, Baker-Gordon Phenol, and Dermabrasion: A Comparative Clinical and Histologic Study of Cutaneous Resurfacing in a Porcine Model," *Archives of Dermatology* 132:4 (April 1996): 469–71; M. T. Speyer et al., "Erythema after Cutaneous Laser Resurfacing Using a Porcine Model," *Archives of Otolaryngology: Head & Neck Surgery* 124:9 (September 1998): 1008–13. See also "IAF Hairless Guinea Pig," *Charles River Associates*, http://www.criver.com/products-services/basic-research/find-a-model/iaf-hairless-guinea-pig-(1); Shayne C. Gad, ed., *Animal Models in Toxicology*, 2nd edition (Boca Raton, FL: Taylor & Francis, 2007), chaps. 5

and 10; Mark A. Suckow et al., *The Laboratory Rabbit, Guinea Pig, Hamster, and Other Rodents* (London: Elsevier, 2012); L. M. Panepinto et al., "The Yucatan Miniature Pig as a Laboratory Animal," *Laboratory Animal Science* 28:3 (June 1978): 308–13; Roy Forster, "Minipig Use in Safety Assessments during Drug Development," *American College of Toxicology,* http://www.actox.org/meetCourses/Webinar_Forster_Minipigs.pdf; J. L. Estrada et al., "Successful Cloning of the Yucatan Minipig Using Commercial/Occidental Breeds as Oocyte Donors and Embryo Recipients," *Cloning and Stem Cells* 10:2 (June 2008): 287–96.

12. Grevelink et al., "Lasers," 2901; Noah Kawika Weisberg and Steven S. Greenbaum, "Pigmentary Changes after Alexandrite Laser Hair Removal," *Dermatologic Surgery* 29:4 (2003): 415–19; Suzanne Yee, "Laser Hair Removal in Fitzpatrick Type IV to VI Patients," *Facial Plastic Surgery* 21:2 (2005): 139–44; S. P. R. Lim and S. W. Lanigan, "A Review of the Adverse Effects of Laser Hair Removal," *Laser in Medical Science* 21 (2006): 121–25.

13. Grevelink et al., "Lasers," 2904.

14. Some laser therapists have been accused of prescribing Vicodan, Percoset, and Oxycodone as an incentive for purchasing laser hair removal. See "Blanco Bolanos & Shiri Berg Die from Overdose of Topical Lidocaine-Tetracaine Anesthetic at Two Different Laser Parlor Clinics 2500 Miles Apart," *Boston School of Electrolysis,* April 28, 2005, http://www.boston-schoolofelectrolysis.com/boston-electrolysis-32.html..

15. Grevelink et al., "Lasers" 2904. Topical gels, air coolers, cryogen sprays, and ice packs have all been used to ameliorate unwanted skin damage.

16. Donald W. Shenenberg and Lynn M. Utecht, "Removal of Unwanted Facial Hair," *American Physician* 66:10 (2002): 1907–11, 1913–14.

17. Susanne Astner and R. Rox Anderson, "Skin Phototypes 2003," *Society for Investigative Dermatology,* February 2, 2004, xxx; Thomas B. Fitzpatrick, *Fitzpatrick's Dermatology in General Medicine,* 5th edition (New York: McGraw-Hill), 1999.

18. Participant I, interview with author, September 3, 2009.

19. Eliot F. Battle Jr. and Lori M. Hobbs, "Laser Assisted Hair Removal for Darker Skin Types," *Dermatologic Therapy* 17 (2004): 180; T. Alster et al., "Long Pulsed Nd: YAG Laser Assisted Hair Removal in Pigmented Skin," *Archives of Dermatology* 137 (2001); E. K. Battle et al., "Very Long Pulses (20–200ms) Diode Laser for Hair Removal on All Skin Types," *Lasers in Surgery and Medicine* 12 (Suppl.) (2000); I. Greppi, "Diode Laser Hair Removal of the Black Patient," *Lasers in Surgery and Medicine*

28 (2002): 150–55; R. M. Adrian and K. P. Shay, "800nm Diode Laser Hair Removal in African American Patients: A Clinical and Histological Study," *Journal of Cutaneous Laser Therapy* 2 (2000): 183–90; Natasha Singer, "Treating Skin of Color with Know-How: A New Generation of Dermatologists and Clinics for an Expanding Market," *New York Times*, November 3, 2005, E1.

20. Packaged Facts, "Market Trends: Shaving/Hair Removal Products," Publication ID: LA1097891, 2005, http:www.packagedfacts.com/pub/1097891.html.

21. For fuller treatment of the racialization of perceptions of body hair, see Bessie Rigakos, "Women's Attitudes toward Body Hair and Hair Removal: Exploring Racial Differences in Beauty," Ph.D. diss., Wayne State University, 2004; Susan Bordo, *Unbearable Weight: Feminism, Western Culture, and the Body* (Berkeley: University of California Press, 1993), 253–55.

22. Paul Starr, *The Social Transformation of American Medicine* (New York: Basic Books, 1982), 421; Deborah A. Sullivan, *Cosmetic Surgery: The Cutting Edge of Commercial Medicine in America* (New Brunswick. NJ: Rutgers University Press, 2001), 70.

23. Kayhan Parsi, "International Medical Graduates and US Health Care: A Win/Win or Uneasy Detente," paper delivered at the Southern Association for the History of Medicine and Science 8th Annual Conference, San Antonio, Texas, February 25, 2006; Sullivan, *Cosmetic Surgery*, 70.

24. "Trends and Indicators in the Changing Health Care Market Place," *Kaiser Family Foundation*, 2002, http://www.kff.org/insurance/3161-index.cfm.

25. Roger J. Hollingsworth, *A Political Economy of Medicine: Great Britain and the United States* (Baltimore, MD: John Hopkins University Press, 1986), 108.

26. Sullivan, *Cosmetic Surgery*.

27. Mark Collar (president of Global Pharmaceuticals and Personal Health at Procter & Gamble), cited in "Sponsor Profile," in *Biotech360*, from the *Scientist Magazine* (2007): 66.

28. Jan E. Thomas and Mary K. Zimmerman, "Feminism and Profit in American Hospitals: The Corporate Construction of Women's Health Centers," *Gender & Society* 21:3 (June 2007): 359–83.

29. Participant I, interview with author, September 3, 2009.

30. Sullivan, *Cosmetic Surgery*, 70, 192–93.

31. R. F. Wagner Jr., "Medical and Technical Issues in Office Electrolysis and Thermolysis," *Journal of Dermatologic Surgery and Oncology* 19 (1993):

575–77; R. N. Richards and G. E. Meharg, *Cosmetic and Medical Electrolysis and Temporary Hair Removal: A Practice Manual and Reference Guide*, 2nd edition (Toronto: Medric, 1997); Elise A. Olsen "Methods of Hair Removal," *Journal of American Academy of Dermatology* 40:2 (1999): 143–55; Weisberg and Greenbaum, "Pigmentary Changes," 415.

32. Bruce M. Freedman and Robert V. Earley, "Comparing Treatment Outcomes between Physician- and Nurse-Treated Patients in Laser Hair Removal," *Journal of Cutaneous Laser Therapy* 2:3 (2000): 137–40; "Decision Regarding Laser Devices/Appearance Enhancement Licensees," January 28, 2010, New York State Division of Licensing Services, http://www.dos.ny.gov/licensing/news.html.

33. Kincade, "Alexandrite," 63–64.

34. Gail Garfinkel Weiss, "Adding Ancillaries: Laser Hair Removal," *Medical Economics* 82:21 (2005): 2.

35. Participant I, interview with author, September 3, 2009.

36. Christopher Rowland, "Doctors Target Laser Procedures as New Revenue Source," *Boston Globe*, September 30, 2005, A1.

37. Participant I, interview with author, September 3, 2009.

38. Rowland, "Doctors Target Laser Procedures," A1.

39. Ibid.

40. Originally priced at $995, the Tria's promoters explicitly sought to capitalize on hair removal's position as "the number one use of lasers in medicine today." See Naomi Torres, "Interview with Bob Grove, Co-founder of Tria Beauty," *About.Com*, http://hairremoval.about.com/od/lase1/a/tria-beauty.htm.

41. H. Ray Jalian et al., "Lawsuit Cases Rising for Cutaneous Laser Surgery," *JAMA Dermatology* 149:2 (2013): 188–93; Genevra Pittman, "Laser Surgery Injuries Spurring More Lawsuits against Non-Doctors," *NBC News*, October 16, 2013.

42. Participant I, interview with author, September 3, 2009.

43. gina in East Bay, November 20, 2011, *RealSelf.com*, http://www.realself.com/review/berkeley-laser-hair-removal-simple-process-proves-life-changing. It should be noted that most of the online forums devoted to evaluations of laser hair removal (including those found at *RealSelf.com*) are sponsored in part or in full by people with direct financial interests in the practice.

44. zippyty, July 12, 2011, *RealSelf.com*, http://www.realself.com/review/clear-water-fl-laser-hair-removal-laser-review-painful.

45. FinallyFree, September 17, 2010, *RealSelf.com*, http://www.realself.com/

review/st-louis-laser-hair-removal-worth1.

46. kristelle123, August 11, 2009, *RealSelf.com*, http://www.realself.com/re-view/Laser-hair-removal-Burned-removing-hair; Isabelle685, April 27, 2014, *RealSelf.com*, http://www.realself.com/review/allentown-pa-dont-laser-hair-removal-places-without-hair-places-without-visible.

47. Noah Kawika Weisberg and Steven S. Greenbaum, "Pigmentary Changes after Alexandrite Laser Hair Removal," *Dermatologic Surgery* 29:4 (2003): 418; A. Alajlan et al., "Paradoxical Hypertrichosis after Laser Epilation," *Journal of the American Academy of Dermatology* 53:1 (July 2005): 85–88.

48. M. Hussain et al., "Laser-Assisted Hair Removal in Asian Skin: Efficacy, Complications, and the Effect of Single versus Multiple Treatments," *Dermatologic Surgery* 29:3 (2003): 249, 254.

49. Freedman and Earley, "Comparing Treatment Outcomes," 138.

50. Weisberg and Greenbaum, "Pigmentary Changes," 418.

51. Ibid. See also A. T. Hasan et al., "Solar-Induced Postinflammatory Hyper-pigmentation after Laser Hair Removal," *Dermatologic Surgery* 25 (1999): 113–15; C. H. Garcia et al., "Alexandrite Hair Removal Is Safe for Fitzpat-rick Skin Types IV-VI," *Dermatologic Surgery* 26 (2000): 130–34; H. H. Chan et al., "An *In Vivo* Study Comparing the Efficacy and Complications of Diode Laser and Long-Pulsed Nd: YAG Laser in Hair Removal of Chi-nese Patients," *Dermatologic Surgery* 27 (2001): 950–54; V. B. Campos et al., "Ruby Laser Removal: Evaluation of Long-Term Efficacy and Side Ef-fects," *Lasers in Surgery and Medicine* 26 (2000): 177–85; K. Toda et al., "Alternation of Racial Differences in Melanosome Distribution in Human Epidermis after Exposure to Ultraviolet Light," *Nature: New Biology* 236 (1972): 143–45.

52. Weisberg and Greenbaum, "Pigmentary Changes," 417.

53. Abigail Leichman, "Red Flags for Those with Skin of Color: When It Comes to Safe Topical Treatments, It Is a Matter of Black and White," *Record* (Bergen County, New Jersey), December 27, 2005.

54. Andrea James, "Laser Hair Removal Injuries to Dark Skin," http://www.youtube.com/watch?v=XpZcBKdBoVg.

55. *Estelle v. Gamble*, 429 U.S. 97 (1976); *Helling v. McKinney*, 509 U.S. 25 (1993).

56. Will O'Bryan, "Gender in Virginia: Transgender Inmate Sues for Surgery," *MetroWeekly*, June 16, 2011, http://www.metroweekly.com/news/?ak=6349&amp&amphttp://www.metroweekly.com/news/?ak=6349&amp& Jordan Gwendolyn Davis, "Trans Woman in Mass Prison Must Receive Laser, Conservative Federal Judge Says,"

Feministing.com, February 15, 2012, http://community.feministing. com/2012/02/15/trans-woman-in-mass-prison-must-receive-laser-con-servative-federal-judge-says; Nathaniel Penn, "Should This Inmate Get a State-Financed Sex Change Operation?" *New Republic*, October 30, 2013, http://www.newrepublic.com/article/115335/sex-change-prison-inmate-michelle-kosilek-should-we-pay.

57. "Hair Removal Statistics from American Laser Centers," June 24, 2008, *Skin Care and Beauty News*, http://www.skincareblog.net/2008/06/24/hair-removal-statistics-from-american-laser-centers.

NOTES TO CHAPTER 9

1. "U.S. Biotech Revenues, 1992–2001," *Biotechnology Industrial Organization*, http://www.bio.org/ataglance/bio/2002101rva.asp; "The Human Genome," *Nature*, February 15, 2001; "The Human Genome," *Science*, February 16, 2001; "Building on the DNA Revolution," *Science*, April 11, 2003; "Double Helix at 50," *Nature*, April 24, 2003; Raymond A. Zilinskas and Peter J. Balint, eds., *The Human Genome Project and Minority Communities: Ethical, Social, and Political Dilemmas* (Westport, CT: Praeger, 2001); Kevin Davies, *Cracking the Genome: Inside the Race to Unlock Human DNA* (New York: Free Press, 2001); James Shreeve, *The Genome War: How Craig Venter Tried to Capture the Code of Life and Save the World* (New York: Knopf, 2004).

2. See, for example, Maxwell J. Mehlman and Kristen M. Rabe, "Any DNA to Declare? Regulating Offshore Access to Genetic Enhancement," *American Journal of Law and Medicine* 28:2/3 (2002): 179–204; Michael J. Sandel, *The Case against Perfection: Ethics in the Age of Genetic Engineering* (Cambridge, MA: Harvard University Press, 2007); Jenny Reardon, *Race to the Finish: Identity and Governance in an Age of Genomics* (Princeton, NJ: Princeton University Press, 2005); Susan M. Lindee, *Moments of Truth: Genetic Disease in American Culture* (Baltimore, MD: John Hopkins University Press, 2005); Troy Duster, *Backdoor to Eugenics*, 2nd edition (New York: Routledge, 2003); Alan H. Goodman et al., *Genetic Nature/Culture: Anthropology and Science beyond the Two-Culture Divide* (Berkeley: University of California Press, 2003); Keith Wailoo et al., *Genetics and the Unsettled Past: The Collision of DNA, Race, and History* (New Brunswick, NJ: Rutgers University Press, 2012); Arthur Frank, "Emily's Scars: Surgical Shapings, Technoluxe, and Bioethics," *Hasting Center Report* 34:2 (2004) 18–29.

3. Nikolas Rose, *The Politics of Life Itself: Biomedicine, Power, and Subjectivity in the Twenty-first Century* (Princeton, NJ: Princeton University Press, 2006), 11–12; Adele E. Clarke, Janet Shim, Laura Mamo, Jennifer Fosket, and Jennifer Fishman, eds., *Biomedicalization: Technoscience, Health, and Illness in the U.S.* (Durham, NC: Duke University Press, 2010), 68–70; Abby Lippman, "Led (Astray) by Genetic Maps: The Cartography of the Human Genome and Health Care," *Social Science and Medicine* 35:12 (1992): 1469-76.

4. "GeneLink and Arch Personal Care Products Present 'Genetic Skin Care' Products at International Cosmetic Expo," *Business Wire*, February 20, 2003; GeneLink Inc., "Arch Personal Care Products and GeneLink to Begin Marketing 'Genetic' Skin Care Kit and Formulations to Marketers and Manufacturers for the Personal Care and Cosmetic Industries," Press Release, February 30, 2003; R. Baran and H. I. Maibach, eds., *Cosmetic Dermatology* (London: Martin Dunitz, 1994); P. Elsner and H. I. Maibach, eds., *Cosmeceuticals* (New York: Marcel Dekker, 2000); Kostas Kostarelos, "Biotechnology Impacting Cosmetic Science: Altering the Way Cosmetics Are Perceived," *Cosmetics and Toiletries* 117:1 (2002): 34–38. Also see Amy Newburger and Arthur Caplan, "Taking Ethics Seriously in Cosmetic Dermatology," *Archives of Dermatology* 142:2 (2006): 1641–42.

5. "RNA: Really New Advances," *Economist*, June 14, 2007, 87–89; "Eyeing 11B Hair Removal Market, Sirna Acquires Skinetics," *RNAiNews*, December 10, 2004.

6. On the prevalence of hair removal, see Debra Herbenick et al., "Pubic Hair Removal among Women in the United States: Prevalence, Methods, and Characteristics," *Journal of Sexual Medicine* 7(2010): 3322-3330.; Michael Boroughs, Guy Cafri, and J. Thompson, "Male Body Depilation: Prevalence and Associated Features of Body Hair Removal," *Sex Roles* 52:9–10 (May 2005): 637–44.

7. Participant G, interview with author, March 17, 2010.

8. Participant B, interview with author, July 17, 2009.

9. Freeman Dyson, "Our Biotech Future," *New York Review of Books*, July 19, 2007. See also Arthur Caplan, "Commentary: Improving Quality of Life Is a Morally Important Goal for Gene Therapy," *Human Gene Therapy* 17 (December 2006): 1164.

10. Richard Robinson, "RNAi Therapeutics: How Likely, How Soon?" *PLoS Biology* 2:1 (January 2004): 18–20.

11. J. Couzin, "Small RNAs Make Big Splash," *Science*, December 20, 2002; Kristen Philipkoski, "Next Big Thing in Biotech: RNAi," *Wired*, Novem-

ber 20, 2003; D. Stripp, "Biotech's Billion Dollar Breakthrough: A Technology Called RNAi Has Opened the Door to Major New Drugs," *Fortune*, May 12, 2003.

12. A. Fire et al., "Potent and Specific Genetic Interference by Double-Stranded RNA in *Caenorhabditis Elegans*," *Nature* 391 (1998): 806–11; "RNA: Really New Advances."

13. Richard A. Strum et al., "Human Pigmentation Genes: Identification, Structure, and Consequences of Polymorphic Variation," *Gene* 277:1–2 (2001); "On the Trail of the Gene for Extreme Hairiness," *Boston Globe*, June 1, 1995, A3; Luis E. Figuera et al., "Mapping of the Congenital Generalized Hypertrichosis Locus to Chromosome Xq24-Q27.1," *Nature Genetics* 10 (1995); P. E. Valverde et al., "Variants of the Melanocyte-Stimulating Hormone Receptor Genes Are Associated with Red Hair and Fair Skin in Humans," *Nature Genetics* 11 (1995).

14. Thomas Andl et al., "The miRNA-Processing Enzyme Dicer Is Essential for the Morphogenesis and Maintenance of Hair Follicles," *Current Biology* 6:10 (2006); D. Garcia Cruz et al., "Inherited Hypertrichosis," *Clinical Genetics* 61:5 (2002): 321–29; B. A. Morgan, "Upending the Hair Follicle," *Nature Genetics* 38:3 (2006).

15. This chapter is based on six months of ethnographic study of four internet discussion boards and twenty-five tape-recorded, transcribed, semistructured interviews. Per the requirements of the Bates College Institutional Review Board, all participants' identities are concealed.

16. The technical challenges involved in making an effective RNAi-based hair remover are myriad. The formulation must be able to be produced at a reasonable cost; to reach target cells before being excreted, degraded by nucleases, or absorbed by other tissues; to penetrate the intended cells; and to exert an effect on those targets without serious toxicity. Most industry leaders agree that affordable manufacturing is the most readily manageable of these challenges. The more significant obstacles involve delivery: getting the RNA to the relevant cells, persuading those cells to take it up, and delivering siRNAs to their intracellular targets without adverse effects. RNAi hair removal faces the additional barrier of getting a large molecule through the outer layer of the epidermis (the stratum corneum) and down the rather long hair shaft. As one former company executive recalled, "[I]t just didn't work. And we really tried everything that we could think of. Everything that was out there. We tried everything that people suggest. Came up with a lot of our own things. . . . And we weren't able to get in there" (Participant B, interview with author, July 17, 2009). To date, re-

searchers have not found a feasible, reliable way to deliver hair-retarding siRNAs to their targets in the living body. For further discussion of the challenges of RNAi delivery, see Enrico Mastrobattista, Wim E. Hennink, and Raymond M. Schieffelers, "Delivery of Nucleic Acids," *Pharmaceutical Research* 24:8 (August 2007): 1561–63.

17. Patricia G. Engasser and Howard I. Maibach, "Cosmetics and Skin Care in Dermatologic Practice," in *Fitzpatrick's Dermatology in General Medicine*, 5th ed., vol. 2, ed. Irwin M. Freedberg et al. (New York: McGraw Hill, 1999), 2778–82.

18. Participant B, interview with author, July 17, 2009.

19. Participant G, interview with author, March 17, 2010.

20. Cynthia Enloe, *Seriously! Investigating Crashes and Crises as if Women Mattered* (Berkeley: University of California Press, 2013), 1–18. On relational constitution more generally, see Judith Butler, *Bodies That Matter: On the Discursive Limits of "Sex"* (New York: Routledge, 1993).

21. Participant D, interview with author, September 3, 2009. See also ShawnTe Pierce, "Botox and Cerebral Palsy: FDA Findings for This Unapproved Use of Botox," *Suite101.com*, May 15, 2009, http://physical-disabilities.suite101.com/article.cfm/botox_and_cerebral_palsy; "Look Who's Growing Longer, Fuller, Darker Lashes," *Latisse*, http://www.latisse.com.

22. The concept of "lifestyle drugs" merits a historical study of its own. It seems worth mentioning here that the word "lifestyle" entered the English language only in 1915, just as x-ray hair removal was taking off. The *Oxford English Dictionary* lists 1982 as the first reference to "lifestyle drugs."

23. Participant B, interview with author, July 17, 2009.

24. Ibid.

25. Ibid.

26. Participant E, interview with author, November 27, 2009.

27. For a tidy summary of the process, see Natasha Singer, "Sure, It's Treatable: But Is It a Disorder?" *New York Times*, December 13, 2009, 4.

28. Adele E. Clarke and colleagues make a compelling case for the development of a distinct process of "biomedicalization"; I maintain use of the term "medicalization" here for clarity's sake. See their original publication, "Biomedicalization: Technoscientific Transformations of Health, Illness, and U.S. Biomedicine," *American Sociological Review* 68 (April): 161–94. Also see Ilana Löwy, "Historiography of Biomedicine: 'Bio,' 'Medicine,' and in Between," *Isis*, March 2011, 116–22; Peter Conrad, *The Medicalization of Society: On the Transformation of Human Conditions into Treatable Disorders* (Baltimore, MD: Johns Hopkins University Press, 2007); Jona-

than M. Metzl and Rebecca M. Herzig, "Medicalization in the 21st Century: An Introduction," *Lancet*, March 24, 2007, 697–98; and Anne E. Figert and Susan E. Bell, "Gender and the Medicalization of Healthcare," in *The Handbook of Gender and Healthcare*, ed. Ellen Kuhlmann and Ellen Annandale (New York: Palgrave, 2012), 107–22.

29. Participant B, interview with author, July 17, 2009.

30. Ibid.

31. Participant O, interview with author, August 10, 2009.

32. Participant E, interview with author, November 27, 2009.

33. Participant B, interview with author, July 17, 2009.

34. Participant D, interview with author, September 3, 2009.

35. Participant H, interview with author, January 29, 2010.

36. Participant D, interview with author, September 3, 2009, referring to L. Parks et al., "The Importance of Skin Disease as Assessed by 'Willingness to Pay,'" *Journal of Cutaneous Medicine including Surgery* 7:5 (September–October 2003): 369–71.

37. Anat Keinan et al., "Capitalizing on the Underdog Effect," *Harvard Business Review* 88: 11 (November 2010): 32.

38. Rhonda L. Rundel, "A New Name in Skin Care: Johns Hopkins," *Wall Street Journal*, April 5, 2006, B1; Alex Kuczynski, *Beauty Junkies: Inside Our $15 Billion Obsession with Cosmetic Surgery* (New York: Doubleday, 2006); "Clinique Announces Groundbreaking Collaboration with Weill Cornell Department of Dermatology," *Cornell Dermatology*, http://www.cornelldermatology.com/abo_us/new_eve.html?name1=News+and+Events&type1=2Active; Newburger and Caplan, "Taking Ethics Seriously," 1641.

39. Participant D, interview with author, September 3, 2009.

40. "Eyeing $11B Hair Removal Market, Sirna Acquires Skinetics," *RNAiNews*, December 10, 2004; Participant B, interview with author, July 17, 2009.

41. On the role of reputation, trust, and conviviality in contemporary academic and commercial research, see Steven Shapin, *The Scientific Life: A Moral History of a Late Modern Vocation* (Chicago: University of Chicago Press, 2008).

42. Participant W, interview with author, April 8, 2010.

43. Participant G, interview with author, March 17, 2010.

44. Participant R, interview with author, June 25, 2010.

45. Participant B, interview with author, July 17, 2009.

46. See "Quest PharmaTech Announces Second Quarter Results," *Quest Pharmatech, Inc.*, September 15, 2009, http://micro.newswire.ca/release.

cgi?rkey=1709154436&view=43406-0&Start=0&htm=0.

47. Dee Fahey, "Re. Sirna Update," April 26, 2012, *HairTell*, http://www. hairtell.com/forum/ubbthreads.php/topics/98187/Re_Sirna_Update. html#Post98187.

48. Eddy, "Re: Quest pharmatech," October 20, 2006, *HairTell*, http://www. hairtell.com/forum/ubbthreads.php/topics/33295/2.html.

49. Baron, "Re: Quest pharmatech," December 6, 2006, *HairTell*, http://www.hairtell.com/forum/ubbthreads.php/topics/33295/3.html.

50. Participant B, interview with author, July 17, 2009.

NOTES TO THE CONCLUSION

1. The paradox that the expansion of liberal rights of self-governance for privileged Americans (able-bodied, white, male) has nearly always been accompanied by corresponding restrictions on the "selfhood" of others has been charted by several historians. See Amy Dru Stanley, *From Bondage to Contract: Wage Labor, Marriage, and the Market in the Age of Slave Emancipation* (Cambridge: Cambridge University Press, 1998); Eric Foner, *The Story of American Freedom* (New York: Norton, 1998); Barbara Y. Welke, *Law and the Borders of Belonging in the Long-Nineteenth-Century United States* (Cambridge: Cambridge University Press, 2010).

2. Michel Foucault, "The Ethics of the Concern for Self as a Practice of Freedom," in *Ethics: Subjectivity and Truth*, vol. 1, ed. Paul Rabinow (New York: New Press, 1997), 283; and "'*Omnes et Singulatim*': Toward a Critique of Political Reason," in *Power*, vol. 3, ed. James D. Faubion (New York: New Press, 2000), 311.

3. Darius Rejali, *Torture and Democracy* (Princeton, NJ: Princeton University Press, 2007).

4. Scholars taking such a "Foucauldian" approach to body modification include (but are by no means limited to) Alan Petersen, "Governmentality, Critical Scholarship, and Medical Humanities," *Journal of Medical Humanities* 24:3–4 (2003): 192; Victoria Pitts-Taylor, "Medicine, Governmentality, and Biopower in Cosmetic Surgery," in *Legal, Medical, and Cultural Regulation of the Body*, ed. Stephen W. Smith and Ronan Deazley (Farnham, England: Ashgate, 2009); Cressida J. Hayes, *Self-Transformations: Foucault, Ethics, and Normalized Bodies* (Oxford: Oxford University Press, 2007); Suzanne Fraser, *Cosmetic Surgery, Gender, and Culture* (New York: Palgrave Macmillan, 2003); and Alexander Edmonds, *Pretty Modern:*

Beauty, Sex, and Plastic Surgery in Brazil (Durham, NC: Duke University Press, 2010).

5. For a helpful summary of critiques of stratified enhancement, see Carl Elliott, *Better Than Well: American Medicine Meets the American Dream* (New York: Norton, 2003). Also see Paul Farmer, *Pathologies of Power: Health, Human Rights, and the New War on the Poor* (Berkeley: University of California Press, 2003), esp. 174; Carl Elliott, "Enhancement Technology," in *Readings in the Philosophy of Technology*, ed. David Kaplan (Lanham, MD: Rowman and Littlefield, 2009), 373–79; and Adele Clarke et al., "Biomedicalization: A Theoretical and Substantive Introduction," in Adele Clarke et al., eds., *Biomedicalization: Technoscience, Health, and Illness in the U.S.* (Durham, NC: Duke University Press, 2010), esp. 29.

6. My thinking about temporal and geographical distributions of suffering is particularly indebted to two texts. First, Rob Nixon's related call for increased attention to "slow violence," which he defines as violence that "occurs gradually and out of sight, a violence of delayed destruction that is dispersed across time and space, an attritional violence that is typically not viewed as violence at all. . . neither spectacular nor instantaneous, but rather incremental and accretive, its calamitous repercussions playing out across a range of temporal scales." See Rob Nixon, *Slow Violence and the Environmentalism of the Poor* (Cambridge, MA: Harvard University Press, 2011), 2. Second, Gabrielle Hecht's account of the geographical and colonial dimensions of "nuclearity," and related understandings of "security." See Gabrielle Hecht, *Being Nuclear: Africans and the Global Uranium Trade* (Cambridge, MA: MIT Press, 2012).

7. Powerful social movements are springing up to rectify this problem. I would note here the crucial contributions of Health Care without Harm (http://www.noharm.org), working to bring environmental justice and sustainability to health care; the Campaign for Safe Cosmetics (http://www.safecosmetics.org), a coalitions of workers' rights, environmental, public health, and consumer groups focused on the beauty industry; and the Basel Action Network (http://www.ban.org), which confronts the affluent world's devastating, and increasing, dumping of electronic waste into poor communities.

8. On the importance of attending to "boring things," see Susan Leigh Star, "The Ethnography of Infrastructure," *American Behavioral Scientist* 43:3 (1999): 377–91.

9. For further discussion, see Thomas Lemke, *Biopolitics: An Advanced Introduction* (New York: New York University Press, 2011).

10. As Peter Miller and Nikolas Rose point out, expertise is the glue that aligns "personal choices with the ends of government." See "Political Power beyond the State," *British Journal of Sociology* 43:2 (1992): 285. For more on the role of experts and expertise in neoliberal self-governance, see Miller and Rose, "On Therapeutic Authority: Psychoanalytic Expertise under Advanced Liberalism," *History of the Human* Sciences 7:3 (1994): 29–64; and Rose, *The Politics of Life Itself* (Princeton, NJ: Princeton University Press, 2007), esp. 6.

11. Donna J. Haraway, *When Species Meet* (Minneapolis: University of Minnesota Press, 2008), 297. On the resulting need to place our own meaning making practices at the core of contemporary ethics and politics, see Rosalind Pollack Petchesky, "The Body as Property: A Feminist Re-vision," in *Conceiving the New World Order: The Global Politics of Reproduction*, ed. Faye D. Ginsberg and Rayna Rapp (Berkeley: University of California Press, 1995), 387–406.

12. Norman O. Brown, *Love's Body* (Berkeley: University of California Press, 1966), 155.

Index

abjection, 200n11, 261n64

abortion parlors, 59, 95, 217n18

adverse health affects: of depilatories, 47–49, 54, 79–80, 219n36, 234n26, 242n4; of laser hair removal, 156–158, 166, 168–169, 263n15; personal injury claims, 96, 164, 169, 240n95; of abrasives, 79; of waxing, 79, 137, 148–149, 150–151; of x-ray hair removal, 87–88, 96–97, 239n89. *See also* pain; regulatory oversight; suffering

advertising/marketing: branding, 50, 180; class mobility and, 90–95; depilatories, 40–43, 49–51, 52–54; direct-to-consumer, 159–60; gender and, 76, 78–79, 92, 167; home hair removal, 164, 266n40; impact on pubic hair removal, 258n32; laser hair removal, 153–154, 158, 159–160, 164–169; Orientalism and, 50–54; race and, 40, 76, 78–79, 90, 92–93, 158; scientific advancement and, 89–90; of shaving, 123–126; x-ray hair removal, 89–95, 96, 239n81

African Americans, 22, 128, 203n32, 204n35. *See also* enslaved peoples

age: genital hair removal and, 135–137, 145; hairiness and, 10–11, 28, 67, 71, 113–114, 127, 145, 167, 179; hypertrichosis diagnosis/treatment and, 67; laser hair removal and, 154

Allergan, Inc., 177, 180

Alley, Kirstie, 139

al-Qahtani, Mohammed, 2

al-Sharbi, Ghassan Abdullah, 2

American Dermatological Association, 65–66

American Laser Centers, 167

animals: animal glands, 101–103, 242n13; animality, 12–13, 27, 64–65, 73–74, 253n67; animal models/testing, 155, 182, 190; animal rights, 133–134, 182, 253n67, 256n19; evolution and, 12–13, 56–58, 62–63; excessive human hair and, 12–13, 64, 73–74, 253n67; gorillas, 61–63; sexual selection and, 59–60; tannery work, 221n47; unhairing for meat production, 44–47, 146

anthropology, 32–33, 69

Antonioni, Michelangelo, 141

Apess, William, 22–23

Arden, Elizabeth, 43

Aristotle, 100

Atkinson's depilatory, 42–43

Avon, Inc., 172

About the Author

REBECCA M. HERZIG is Christian A. Johnson Professor of Interdisciplinary Studies and Chair of the Program in Women and Gender Studies at Bates College. Her previous work includes *Suffering for Science: Reason and Sacrifice in Modern America* (2005) and, with Evelynn Hammonds, *The Nature of Difference: Sciences of Race in the United States from Jefferson to Genomics* (2009). She lives in Lewiston, Maine.

Biopolitics: Medicine, Technoscience,
and Health in the 21st Century
General Editors: Monica J. Casper and Lisa Jean Moore

Missing Bodies: The Politics of Visibility
Monica J. Casper and Lisa Jean Moore

Against Health: How Health Became the New Morality
Edited by Jonathan M. Metzl and Anna Kirkland

*Is Breast Best? Taking on the Breastfeeding Experts and the New High Stakes of
Motherhood*
Joan B. Wolf

Biopolitics: An Advanced Introduction
Thomas Lemke

The Material Gene: Gender, Race, and Heredity after the Human Genome Project
Kelly E. Happe

Cloning Wild Life: Zoos, Captivity, and the Future of Endangered Animals
Carrie Friese

Eating Drugs: Psychopharmaceutical Pluralism in India
Stefan Ecks

Phantom Limb: Amputation, Embodiment, and Prosthetic Technology
Cassandra S. Crawford

Heart-Sick: The Politics of Risk, Inequality, and Heart Disease
Janet K. Shim

Plucked: A History of Hair Removal
Rebecca M. Herzig